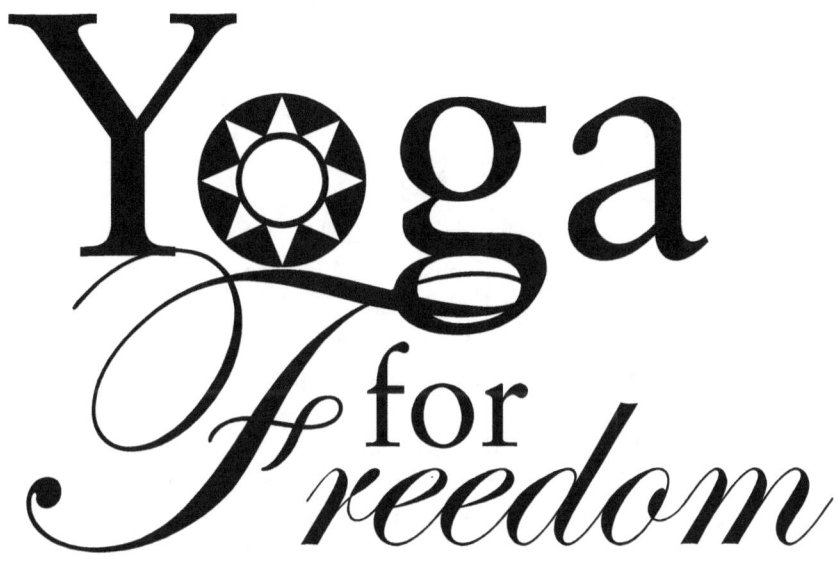

Sivaroshan Sahathevan

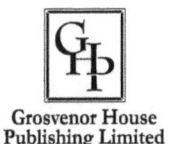

Grosvenor House
Publishing Limited

All rights reserved
Copyright © Sivaroshan Sahathevan, 2025

The right of Sivaroshan Sahathevan to be identified as the author of this work has been asserted in accordance with Section 78 of the Copyright, Designs and Patents Act 1988

The book cover is copyright to Sivaroshan Sahathevan

This book is published by
Grosvenor House Publishing Ltd
Link House
140 The Broadway, Tolworth, Surrey, KT6 7HT.
www.grosvenorhousepublishing.co.uk

This book is sold subject to the conditions that it shall not, by way of trade or otherwise, be lent, resold, hired out or otherwise circulated without the author's or publisher's prior consent in any form of binding or cover other than that in which it is published and without a similar condition including this condition being imposed on the subsequent purchaser.

A CIP record for this book
is available from the British Library

ISBN 978-1-83615-146-3
eBook ISBN 978-1-83615-147-0

DISCLAIMER

Yoga practice

Yoga is a wonderful, diverse exploration of mind, body and spirit; it has many benefits, hence its longevity.

That said, please use your intuition and discernment when practising the kriyās, postures and meditations offered in this publication.

If you are at all uncertain of your fitness to practice at a physical, mental or emotional level, please consult a suitably qualified medical professional before you undertake any of the practices.

The author shall not be held liable for any injury, be it physical or mental, that arises from practice and that you practice by your own free will and at your own risk.

CONTENTS

Disclaimer	iii
Why this book?	vii
Who is this book for?	viii
My background	ix
Kriyā	xii
Leela	xiii
A note on the origins of yoga and kriyā	xiv
Advaita Vedanta	xv
Meditation	xvi
Pranayama	xvii
Mantra	xix
Just sitting and being	xx
Chakras, nadis, kundalini and aura	1
Bandhas	5
Basics of practice	7
Emergence	11
Blue sky	15
Giving it to source	19
Developing steadiness	23
Return to the essence	27
Crack open the shell	32
Heaven to earth	37
Stillness is the new norm	43
Essence of expression	47
Power to the heart	52
Standing steady in expansion – let it come to you	56
Embracing one's strength	60
Bring the light – preparing the body for soul action	64
Steady the ship	68
Passion for Divine	73
Clean out!	78
Conclusion	82
About the author	83

WHY THIS BOOK?

This book started off with requests from students who wanted to practice the unique kriyās that I instructed in class. So the idea for the book was born.

Yet when I put pen to paper, things started to flow a little differently. Something deeper started to present itself; perhaps it was an expression of my personal evolution or maybe even inspiration from 'mother yoga herself'?

My first experience of kriyā was pure, innocent, transformational and evocative. It brought vitality to my body, while touching something far more important, which at the time I did not have words for.

Fast forward almost two decades and I still can't explain it, but maturity has shown me that explanation can be overrated and that sometimes one simply just needs to share.

WHO IS THIS BOOK FOR?

Yoga often calls when 'something's up'.

It can shine a light on our blind spots, helping us reach a deeper understanding of our lives.

If you are curious about what can be revealed through the power of yoga, then this book is for you.

Yoga is a vast subject; we only need to visit our local yoga studio to see various different expressions. Writing this book has been a challenge simply to decide what to include and not include. In the end I decided to keep it relatively simple.

It has been written for all levels, though some experience of practice would be advantageous before undertaking the kriyās in this book.

MY BACKGROUND

How far back does one go to identify the beginning? In some sense it is impossible. Some say the path is written; others say it is carved by our will!

Like most things it probably sits somewhere in between.

My spiritual explorations would be met with raised eyebrows by some and a knowing smile by others, depending on when and where our life paths crossed.

Most of us can relate to this, our life experiences like chapters in a book.

Yet sometimes a shift feels so profound that a chapter shall not suffice; instead a new book must be written. So it was for me.

I use the term *peak experience* to capture those moments that cannot be understood within the library of our intellect or anything else for that matter.

In such moments one is taken out of our known world, into another 'plane', before returning and being left to compute the whole startling episode!

One may never be able to completely understand it, but that does not negate the depth and power of the experience had.

On my quest for truth, understanding – once the panacea of all intellectual investigation – was superseded by something else, best described as a burgeoning intuitive boldness!

The intellect does not normally accept such encroachment lightly and a battle for influence within my mind followed.

Yet, with perseverance my inner landscape started to feel distinctly different; while the battle may not be wholly won, a more refined consciousness has claimed a majority stake.

It is from this place that I share.

One could say that this book represents the insight on the other side of the battle.

I do not profess to be the best or the greatest, only that my intention to share comes from a true place, reflective of my life, my journey and insights.

The 'soul explorer' has always existed in me, but it kicked in forcefully following university and travelling. The question 'What do I do with my life?' became real for the first time and the question of 'my purpose' took centre stage.

It was here that I had a mini cosmic experience, a wisdom from beyond reached towards me and effectively shook me!

I was directed mysteriously to a local WHSmiths (a UK bookstore) to a tiny shelf dedicated to self-help books and I purchased my first book on yoga.

A contract of sorts was formed in that purchase, and the game had begun. The detailed journey from this point on is probably best explained under the cover of another publication but here is a synopsis:

Ever practical, my career path had been ignited, but I was also being guided from the unseen realm. As the years wore on, covert hidden explorations in the world of Yoga and energy healing became more pronounced, finding the light of day firstly in the form of raja yoga, reiki and Buddhist practice. Life choices increasingly were directed into the spiritual dimension. The festive periods no longer in public houses but now in retreats seeking stillness and insight.

As investment in my spiritual will grew, so did the contributions of grace. In one such deep retreat I heard a clear voice in my mind, making it clear that yoga would be my next endeavour.

In a blink of an eye synchronicity brought me to kundalini yoga first popularised in the late 1960s by 3HO and its founder, Yogi Bhajan.

Within this framework I discovered my teacher up in the Alps. I surrendered to a deeper level of personal excavation and the technology of kundalini prepared me physically, mentally and energetically.

This period coincided with an expansion of my exploration into the world of energy healing and the development of my channelling capability.

I became like a sponge, and driven by a thirst to learn, I explored a multitude of energy healing systems and studies to develop my intuitive and psychic ability. It was as if I was riding two galloping horses. Little did I know that the time would come for me to ride my own horse.

Deep insight and visceral, intuitive directness led me to decouple myself from all existing schools and associations. I was in a period of free fall; one could say another chapter was complete.

I landed in a place of self-leadership and deepening commitment to my life path. This book is a result of this.

KRIYĀ

When we seek the edge, we discover that the edge disappears.

That is kriyā.

Kriyā translates as 'complete action'. In the context of yoga – this points to a sequencing of asana, pranayama, mantra and meditation that ignites an elevation of consciousness.

Kriyās are like art; they stand alone in that sense. They may be created by teachers yet they hold long after the teacher has moved to ashes. Just like the painting lives on long after its artist.

Yoga kriyās are, I think, quite like mathematical equations– integers and fractions dancing together with multiples and divisions somehow yielding a specific outcome, but unlike a mathematical equation, the sum is beyond that of its parts! This part of the yogic equation can never be reconciled, a unique factor. Perhaps we can call it divine?

LEELA

We arise from the infinite, and we return to the infinite. That is the way of life and the way of kriyā. Kriyā opens a door to the unknown and invites us to step through.

The energy of kriyā is reflective of the divine play; just as the world has many projections and nuances, so does kriyā.

Leela is the Sanskrit word that is used to describe the play of life; the yogis of old defined the human challenge as navigating this game board of life to return home back to cosmic consciousness.

In fact the enlightened masters of India developed a game of knowledge to help humanity navigate the divine play. In the game one is faced with seventy-two squares or possibilities – each represented by a life quality to be mastered.

On the board itself lie snakes and arrows. Arrows are power-ups that help you ascend the board; snakes work in the reverse, they take you back down to a life lesson not fully mastered and you figure out what was missed.

Kriyās may then be understood in this context: they are practices to help dissolve the samsaras on the game board of life so that one can progress in life with positivity and wisdom. Just like the game board of life, a kriyā can take many shapes; in this way they have the potential to unlock different blocks. How this happens in practice is unique to the individual, a mixture of intention, kriyā and grace.

The kriyās I share have this flavour.

They emerge from an inner resonance, an attenuation to a frequency that guides me in the moment. A feeling, an image, a phrase shows itself and from this the sequence unfolds.

We need but to reach into the purest part of ourselves, and know that is enough; kriyā that arises like this touches the innocence that is in the hearts of all. We are light at our essence – so let's be that.

The kriyās in this publication I share for the purposes of upliftment and elevation. They are taken from the classes I teach, but they also represent my soul, my spirit and commitment.

I hope you enjoy them.

A note on the origins of yoga and kriyā

Yoga is a hugely diverse practice that has continually evolved since its inception thousands of years ago, and shall no doubt continue to evolve. The practices here are simply another piece of an evolutionary arc.

While I feel these kriyās are uniquely creative and hold a certain energy as a result, yoga's tradition is metamorphic, and it feels important to recognise and honour its 'open source' tradition.

Sequences may come together in similar fashion yet have quite different impacts depending on subtle variation, intention, or transmission from a teacher.

That said, the origins of yoga are important. Lineage offers a history, depth and an empowering backstory to our practice in the present. Not all histories unpack uniformly or indeed pleasantly, yet they hold within them the seed of truth that is at the heart of all yoga practice.

The creator of a kriyā (yoga sequence) has impact and value. However, the deep history of yoga, as refined by the ancient rishis (enlightened beings who acted as a conduit for divine wisdom), placed emphasis on the teachings themselves rather than the teacher, hence the authors of the original Hindu texts remain to this day obscure and mysterious.

For our modern times, perhaps meeting in the middle – where we honour yoga's roots and simultaneously make space for its unique individual expression – is a sensible way forward.

ADVAITA VEDANTA

Many years ago, when I was around five years of age, I was sitting by the window not thinking about anything in particular, when I experienced a vast emptiness, which paradoxically also felt supremely alive.

It was accompanied by an almost indescribable sound: a low hum/roar that seemed to emanate from 'beyond'. Its resonance was captivating.

It was scary but not in a horror movie kind of way. I did not feel especially threatened, I just did not know what it was. Then it stopped and life resumed as normal.

It is only now, so many years later, that I would best describe that experience as an expression of non-duality. Such concepts are beautifully encapsulated by Advaita Vedanta, a philosophy from ancient India.

Advaita means 'non-dual' or whole. Vedanta means 'end of the Vedas', which relates to the Upanishads, an ancient text that is located towards the end of a collection of epic sacred books that underpin Hindu culture, known as the Vedas.

The text talks of an all-pervading force – an essence or energy called Brahman. Brahman is the foundation of all creation; it is formless yet from it all forms are created, giving birth to the world of duality, uniqueness and separation that we appear to experience. This world is built around polarities, which gives rise to the experience of highs and lows in life; the lows we may collectively understand as 'suffering'.

Advaita Vedanta points to the true reality (Brahman) that suffuses the infinitely diverse forms of creation. It proposes that our suffering is a consequence of failing to realise this primal truth. If, however, we realise this truth fully and embrace it in our lives, suffering shall cease.

Practicing kriyās helps us to stabilise our awareness, so that we may appreciate the profound yet highly subtle truths inherent within Advaita Vedanta. Kriyā expressed in this way enables us to meet life with consciousness, inviting us to engage with the lessons that we need to grow, transform and liberate ourselves.

MEDITATION

Kriyā you could say is preparation for meditation. If we come back to the essence of the practice meditation is that which takes us home, back to the source. Cultivation of the meditative mind is probably the single most powerful thing we can do in our lifetime. The act of meditation in its many numerous forms has but one ultimate purpose, to realise the truth.

The beauty is, truth is unfolding continually and is relative to our present moment. So meditation is effective wherever or whoever you are. From beginner to lifetime meditator, the practice works to open your unique consciousness.

I see meditation as the art of dislodging the imposter within. This imposter is very clever, often very charming (that's how they get a foothold). But the imposter has one objective: keep control and keep you away from your treasure.

Meditation develops the capacity to shine a light upon the false. The more you meditate the greater your soul light. The dark spaces and hiding places become fewer. The imposter becomes less of an influence as the luminosity of your essence begins to take the driving seat in your life.

In practising kriyā, one aims to be as present as possible, thus evoking a meditative state. In fact the practice of meditation or awareness should be applied to any technique and ideally throughout life.

PRANAYAMA

Pranayama means control of the breath. There are numerous pranayama, each of which yields quite different effects. In this publication they largely are either done during a physical exercise or as a practice in their own right.

Below are some of the common breaths used throughout this book. (Please note that these are basic guidelines; readers are advised to attend classes for more detailed instruction and supervision.)

Long deep breathing (LDB) – This sounds obvious but it does require some attention especially if the fundamentals of natural breathing are not yet established. The breath requires the practitioner to be in a relaxed state. Breath is via the nose and directed in the first instance down towards the abdomen; the breath then begins to fill naturally from the bottom up. The exhale begins from the chest area, followed by ribs and finally abdomen.

Breath of fire (BOF) – Often used in postures, this breath is dynamic, it involves a quick inhale and exhale of breath through the nose, in a pumping fashion at a rate of around two to three times a second. The inhale and exhale are the same length of time. Breath of fire is considered as one continual breath. In the beginning it can sometimes feel a challenge as the diaphragm muscles are not yet developed to breathe at that speed. Another common challenge is what is called reverse breathing. This is where inhalation is directed in the first instance into the upper part of the lungs or chest area (instead of to the abdomen, which is considered natural breathing). Applying breath of fire when this fundamental of breathing is not established can result in feeling out of breath very quickly or simply feeling very clunky. If this is the case, one is advised to practice long, deep breathing so that this habit is first established.

Stroke or segmented breathing – This type of breath is classically done through the nose (though the mouth is used in some versions). In this breath a long deep breathing inhale and exhale is divided up into segments: four, eight, ten, twelve and so on. Each segment represents a fraction of a total inhale or exhale. For example, in an 8-stroke breath the inhale would comprise of eight strokes (1/8 sniffs x 8) until the lungs are completely full. This would be followed by eight strokes out until the lungs are completely empty. The practitioner should remain as aware as possible keeping each inhale smooth, clearly defined and with low decibels (if possible)!

Alternate nostril breathing – Breathing through alternate nostrils is a natural process, called the 'nasal cycle', the precise point as to when this occurs for an individual varies. But the yogis knew that specific alternate nostril techniques have a very clear and direct impact on our consciousness. Left nostril breathing is said to be lunar/feminine/intuitive in its nature; breathing through the right nostril is said to activate sun/masculine/vitality. The left nostril affects the right brain; the right nostril, the left brain. Pranayama of this type typically have a balancing or calming effect on the psyche.

Mouth breathing – Can have the effect of feeling very invigorating as more breath is inhaled and exhaled in a shorter period of time. Depending on the type of mouth breath evoked, this can also have a detoxifying effect.

Kumbhaka, breath retention – This is where the breath is held either at the end of the inhale or exhale. Typically used at the end of exercises, but also used in more advanced practices.

There are more sub-variations of breath but this gives the basics.

MANTRA

Nothing moves the heart more emphatically than mantra. It is in some sense the heart of yoga, it has the quality of decoupling you from the mind and can take you on a profound journey of realisation without you even knowing.

The capacity of mantra to dislodge the stubborn aspects of self makes it a very powerful tool for the soul's journey. In this publication I share mantras that have really moved me through my direct experience of them. You will find them referenced directly in the kriyā in which they relate.

JUST SITTING AND BEING

Arguably the most important aspect of meditation. Advaita Vedanta points to a 'non-dualistic' nature as being our true reality. Just sitting and being is sometimes overlooked but in many respects, it is the most powerful thing one can do to uncover the truth of our reality.

Just sitting as the observer, the watcher of mind opens us up to our deepest realisation. It builds a channel towards the aliveness of our soul. One of the tenets of Advaita Vedanta is a requirement for direct experience; this should be held true as it acts as a barometer for our true growth in life.

CHAKRAS, NADIS, KUNDALINI AND AURA

Chakras

The word *chakra*, derived from Sanskrit, means 'spinning wheel'. Its use is commonplace in modern culture with the term now openly discussed in lifestyle magazines and frequently referenced throughout the well-being industry.

It is beyond the scope of this book to go into the chakras in any major detail. The reader is invited to investigate at their own leisure the many resources available on this subject. That said, they are central to how kriyā works and to the kundalini energy itself, so I will touch upon them here.

There are seven principal chakras that run from the base of the spine to the crown of the head. Each of the chakras relate to discernible attributes corresponding to the human condition. The chakras act as interfaces between the physical and energetic worlds. They function to process information and ensure that the attributes defined by the chakra are working optimally.

The challenge is that modern life can significantly impact the function of our chakras, resulting in them moving sluggishly, or spinning too vigorously.

When they are off, we are off! Health, wealth, vitality, relationships, clarity, emotions and so on are all affected.

Nadis

The chakras coexist with the three primary nadis (or energy channels); there are thousands of nadis in the human system (there are said to be seventy-two thousand). One can think of them like telephone lines or electricity cables, transporting information, or energy, from one place to another.

The nadis come from the Hindu system of medicine known as Ayurveda. Of the thousands, there are three primary nadis: ida, pingala and sushumna. Sushumna is the central channel – one may imagine it as aligned with the spine itself. Ida is known as the feminine life force and pingala the masculine.

The classical depiction shows the seven chakras housed like service stations along a motorway. The other primary energy channels, ida and pingala, originate from the first chakra (root, base, muladhara). They are often portrayed as serpents that snake along the sushumna, weaving between the chakras.

The journey of ida and pingala, which take slightly different routes and intersect at certain points, finishes at the nostrils. The pranayama technique of alternative nostril breathing directly effects these nadis.

The practice of kriyās has the impact of balancing, clearing and energising the chakras, as well as removing blockages from the nadis.

Kundalini

Much has been said, and will certainly continue to be said, on kundalini and what exactly it is.

Directly interpreted it means 'coiled' or 'circular'. Classical definitions include: 'The lock of the curl of the beloved' and 'coiled serpent energy'.

The first definition denotes a connection to, or longing for, the purest form of love. The second alludes to a power or potency; the mention of a serpent may illicit mystery, depth, or fear. The word *kundalini* in Sanskrit is defined in feminine form, which points to the cosmic force of 'Shakti', a divine energy that animates and preserves all that is.

The discourses and sacred texts of the past lay out a map of potential discovery. Perhaps something that was lost is within our power to regain, should we wish for it, and indeed earn it.

For me, the kundalini is potency, of the most incredible kind. Packed within this potency is the life force of the universe itself. There is no separation; the sages will have us know that the duality we experience in the form of polarity is an illusion. At our core we are constructed from the same building blocks as the universe itself. The kundalini is a force that allows us to dynamically realise this truth. The wisdom has been forgotten, but now it is steadily being reclaimed. The kundalini, one could say, represents the elevated life force required to turn this from intellectual debate to a realised and lived experience.

Is it love or a powerful serpent to be feared?

Well, the 'love of power' versus the 'power of love' holds true here. Your underlying intention shall probably determine the unfoldment of this mysterious energy.

In the kriyās that I share, the kundalini is acknowledged in a respectful way, approached with humility through first seeking mastery of our chakras and energy channels. In the same way we would welcome a revered guest into our home, we clean up and maintain a humble disposition.

Kriyā in this sense prepares the ground for kundalini and you to meet, like a courtship of sorts. All courtships are different but are more likely to succeed when you take the time to get to know each other.

The sensational phenomenon of the kundalini – and one that people often get confused about – is known as spontaneous kundalini rising. This is when energy shifts from a dormant state into a very active state; one could say someone has woken up the snake. The energy moves in an uncompromising serpentine way along the sushumna, piercing through the chakras, attuning them to higher vibrational form. The fallout that people experience ranges from bliss to pain.

It is worth pointing out that these awakenings are not just related to yoga but can arise from any number of spiritual traditions. They may also be induced by drugs, and some people simply have them spontaneously. In almost all occurrences the heightened state abates over time, with the person left to integrate the unique experiences gained.

In my time of teaching and practice, the gradual invitation to kundalini holds true and strong. Kundalini energy emerges for the vast majority bit by bit as the subtle body develops and grows. One could experience it as energy, insight or feeling good (although sometimes it manifests as feeling not so good)!

In some ways the word kundalini is a little misleading because the energy represents itself as various phenomena of sensations in the physical, mental and emotional spheres.

My advice would be to always return to direct experience. Enquire into it – how do you feel about what shows itself? Sitting with these experiences is gold dust; it is a unique gift earned from your investment in kriyā.

Aura

You have likely heard the saying, 'What you see is what you get'. In terms of aura, what you feel is what you get!

Your aura, in some sense, is your sum total. Informed by the disposition of your chakras and channels, it is your energetic fragrance, or hue.

It is magnetic in nature. Magnets exhibit an invisible force; they can repel or attract. If you were to pass a metal object like an iron rod through a magnetic field, you would generate electricity.

Our aura is like a magnetic field, surrounding our bodies to differing extents. It acts as a gatekeeper, allowing energies in or keeping them out.

Aura photography readings depict an aura as varying tones of the rainbow. Through studying the different colours and tones, one may potentially obtain an insight into the well-being or nature of a person.

So, the aura put simply is the light field that we emit from our bodies, and it represents a lot of what is going on within the subtle universe.

In our world that is wedded to the waves of energies that govern our modern-day needs, the aura needs to be looked after.

Kriyās work on the aura as well as the other components of the energetic anatomy.

BANDHAS

Bandhas are body locks that are utilised in yoga practices.

How they are understood and explained differs greatly, so this is simply one approach. They are not necessary for kundalini yoga to be effective but learning and developing them can enhance the subtlety and depth of practice.

Mula Bandha (*Mulbandh* or root lock) is the most commonly applied lock. It involves a discreet controlled muscular hold of the perineum. Mastering this lock takes awareness and development of the very specific muscles involved.

It can take time to realise the benefits of this lock. However, it can be experienced by beginners with a broader directive to squeeze the muscles of the anus, sex organs and navel. These actions create a consolidation of the energy that is generated during practice.

Mula bandha combined with kumbhaka (holding the breath) encourages a subtle opening to the kundalini energy that exists at the base of the spine. The upward force of mula bandha combined with the downward force of kumbhaka creates an alchemical pressure that facilitates an expression of energy along the spine.

In the practice of a kriyā, Mula Bandha along with kumbhaka is often instructed or initiated to conclude an exercise. For example, on finishing a spinal flex sequence the practitioner is invited to inhale, retain the breath, and apply Mula Bandha, holding for between five to ten seconds, before releasing the breath and muscle contraction. A short rest period normally follows, allowing for stillness so that one can experience the effects of the practice.

Applying Mula Bandha and kumbhaka in this manner can be actioned after every exercise in a kriyā if so desired but engaging the lock after a few of the more energising routines can also be enough. While Mula Bandha may not be applied after every exercise, it is common practice to at least apply kumbhaka for a few seconds.

Jalandhara bandha (neck lock) can optionally be applied for all meditative or seated postures, especially when the physical and energy bodies have been primed through practice. Jalandhara bandha helps to regulate the energy that moves up the central channel (sushumna). It provides a useful containment for energy that can make stillness in meditation easier to come by. It is achieved with subtle repositioning of the head in relation to the neck. The head moves in slightly, maintaining its horizontal plane, as if one is being gently pushed on the chin. The effect is a feeling of slight, but not uncomfortable, constriction at the back of the neck.

Uddiyana bandha (diaphragm lock) is probably the least used of the locks, owing to it being a bit more complicated to apply and having fewer direct applications.

The three locks effectively cover the length of the spine. Mula Bandha directs energy up to the solar plexus, and uddiyana bandha constitutes the hydraulics required to 'take to the skies'. It functions to transition energy from the lower half of the torso to the upper part, which begins with the heart chakra (anahata), located at the chest.

As outlined earlier in the chakra section, the energy that moves during kriyā helps to balance and unblock the energy centres. The diaphragm lock is a lever that can certainly help with this.

Uddiyana bandha is applied with kumbhaka but this time with the breath held out. To execute this correctly the neck lock must be applied to create a vacuum of sorts. With the breath emptied, the diaphragm can be drawn up into the space vacated by the lungs. This has the effect of directing the spinal energy further upward, towards the heart centre and beyond.

As mentioned, uddiyana bandha is not often applied within kriyā, but it is worth mentioning as it is one of the three primary bandhas.

BASICS OF PRACTICE

Fit to practice

Everyone is beautifully unique. As a result, there is no single perfect way to be in a posture. So please find your way in, with dedication and care; doing your best and discovering your edge is a good benchmark for practice.

Kriyā works energetically, so even if you are struggling to be in a pose, finding a way to get close will bring benefits. Intention and awareness are highly effective and will bear results even if the posture does not feel 'perfect'!

Some postures in a kriyā can seem impossible to get into. That was certainly the case for me in the beginning; I came from a sporting background and was inherently stiff. My best advice for challenging postures would be to have a sense of humour and be kind to yourself, both mentally and physically. If you need to use props (see equipment section) please do so.

It can be useful to attend a few kundalini inspired yoga classes prior to practising the kriyās in this book.

If you are in any way unsure about your physical or mental capacity to practice, please consult a medical practitioner.

Centring yourself

Before we engage in yoga, it helps to orientate our practice to our higher nature.

This short process is more powerful than we might expect. In the beginning you may not feel its importance, but on the occasion where you skip the brief ritual of 'tuning in', the effects of its absence will likely be felt.

There are many ways in which this orientation can be achieved, in silence, or through ritual. Great sports people tune in all the time, sometimes in quite strange ways. We can all relate to the process of 'getting into the zone', and yoga is no different.

Currently, my preference is to bring my palms together and chant the 'Om' sound, but I encourage you to find a way of entering your practice that works for you.

Ending each exercise

Kriyās are constructed from individual postures or exercises, but how should they 'flow' when you practice?

In some sense a kriyā is telling a story and how it flows can be managed in different ways, a little like choosing the appropriate punctuation for a piece of writing. There is no single perfect way to end a sequence (especially in classes, where a teacher is considering the energy of the group as a whole). However, a solid and effective way to conclude each exercise is to inhale and hold the breath, with or without applying Mula Bandha (see section on bandhas).

The breath-hold acts as a consolidation or punctuation mark within the sequence, while also providing a segue to a period of stillness and silent introspection. The length of the breath-hold is subjective, depending on the experience of the individual and the exercise directly preceding it. Between five and ten seconds is a good length of time in most cases. If a specific length of hold is required for an exercise it will be included as a distinct instruction.

The space held between exercises in a kriyā is vital. It is a short period of integration that allows transformation to happen. The postures tend to affect the glandular and nervous systems while also activating the chakras (energy centres) and aura (human magnetic field).

The duration of the rest period between each exercise is again subjective, depending on the intensity of the exercise plus the experience and capability of an individual, or group of practitioners, to recover from it. However, a good rule of thumb is thirty to sixty seconds for average intensity exercises and one to two minutes for very intense activity. In the rest period, the practitioner simply sits in easy pose (crossed legs) or lies on their back if the preceding exercise is particularly intense, or the posture is closer to a reclined position.

Savasana/relaxation

Please make time for savasana – it is the fruit of the practice.

Lie back, ideally covered with a shawl or blanket. Try and lie down for the full time, normally around ten minutes.

Bring yourself out of savasana gently, initially moving the toes and fingers, then stretching the arms above the head. Proceed with a cat stretch to the left, and then the right, before you hug the knees into your chest, rocking from side to side, and then along the length of the spine to bring yourself back into easy pose.

Finishing a kriyā

To finish a kriyā, I always recommend a period of just sitting in stillness. The intention behind all your hard work is to cultivate a mind-body-spirit balance that affords you the greatest possibility to touch your own divine nature. At the end of this 'just sitting' period you may wish to offer gratitude for the practice, by placing your hands in prayer pose and bowing your forehead to the ground.

Equipment

Please ensure that you have the adequate attire and equipment to practice. I suggest loose clothing that does not inhibit movement, a yoga mat and a cushion or block. Tightness in the hips and lower back can make sitting cross-legged difficult – a cushion or block helps to lift the hips higher than the knees, so it is easier to sit. A blanket is also useful for relaxation. If you have a bolster this can be helpful for some postures, although it isn't wholly necessary.

The kriyās

Choose one that feels right then practice it.

One approach would be to master your chosen kriyā: practice it day after day until you feel a sense of completion regarding the journey or lesson it is offering you. This style of execution works well if you need support in a life situation. Regularity provides the consistency and vibrational elevation that can make all the difference when moving through life's challenges.

When adopting this approach, be aware of the mind's tendency to want to escape a practice that is 'slaying the ego'. It can be useful during such times to reflect on why you feel you have had enough of the kriyā and wish to stop engaging with it. Take a moment to go deeper and see what arises. Perhaps it's had its time, or maybe things are just starting to get interesting?

Another nice way to practice is to choose intuitively or randomly – just open the book and the kriyā that shows itself is the one to work with. The kriyās I have published here have by and large been selected from the studio classes that I teach. For each I have written a little on the source of their inspiration and included an image that feels relevant. I have found that instinctual insight can have a quality of timelessness that serves us in the future; choosing in this manner helps us to get ourselves out of the way, making us more open to surrender, which is crucial for effective practice.

The exercises have instructions with recommended time durations. If you can follow the maximum times then do so, but if that is not possible start with the shorter times and build up.

If you are pregnant, it is advisable to attend specialist pregnancy yoga classes.

The menstrual cycle is different for many women. A lot of my female colleagues practice yoga while on their cycle and benefit from it. The unwritten rule is to trust your body. If you are unsure, especially if you have a heavy bleed, then avoid inversions and practices that require strong engagement of the core and abdomen. You can substitute such postures with simply sitting, or lying on the back, letting your awareness follow your breath.

Summary

The above is aimed to provide the bare basics for practice, indeed entire books can be written on the subchapters above. The spirit of this book is to practice with lightness and awareness and grow from each experience.

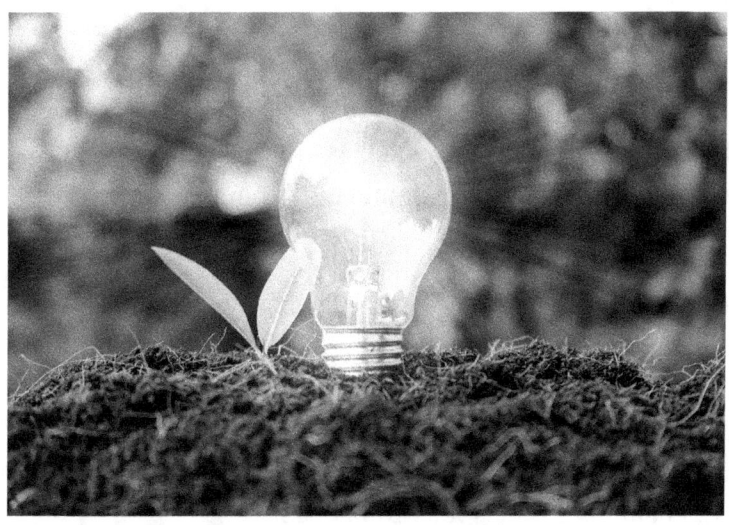

Emergence

True emergence happens when we surrender to authentic expression. There is a jettisoning of weight, a feeling of relief and the experience of joy.

It's a moment that one never forgets, it becomes the barometer for living.

The status quo has competition!

If we allow it to penetrate our lives fully and completely, life shall change. It will become effortless as we hone an instinct that was always there, but rarely used.

As we anchor into this way of being, we may ask ourselves, 'Why did we not do this sooner?'

We understand that it is more than just a personal choice but that it has an impact far deeper and wide reaching.

All of our network with which we engage are the first recipients.

Then there are the strangers who come into our presence. They may not be able to put a finger on it but they feel it.

You become detonators of change, contributors to an increasing frequency on the planet.

1. **Arm pumps.** Begin seated, fingers interlaced, arms extended straight out ahead. Inhale forcefully and equally forcefully bring the arms up, exhale, bring the hands down. Continue this dynamic movement of the arms. For 2–3 min.

   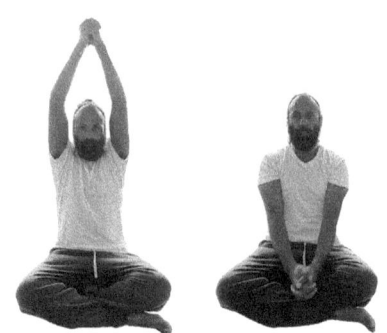

2. **Spinal flexes, big toes.** Sit in easy pose. Hold on to the fleshy part of the big toes with the thumbs, begin to flex the spine. Inhale forward, exhale back for 2–3 min.

   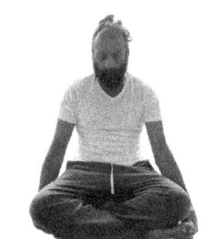 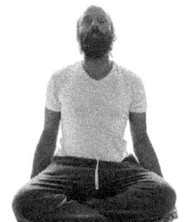

3. **Life nerve stretch.** Sit with the legs out straight, reach forward and grab the toes, in this position exhale and fold forward from the waist. Inhale, return back up, move without forcing while keeping the shoulders relaxed. Move quickly for 2–3 min.

   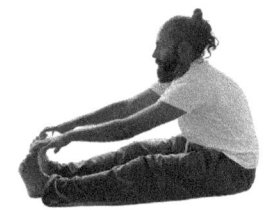 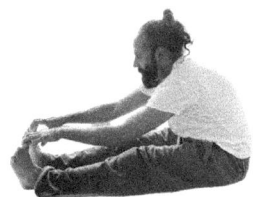

4. **Individual leg stretch with breath of fire.** Extend the right leg straight, left foot into right thigh, breath of fire, 1–2 min. Then switch legs and repeat 1–2 min.

   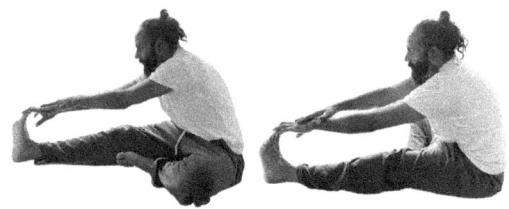

5. **On back static butterfly.** Right hand on chest, left hand on abdomen. Long deep yogic breathing for 1–2 min. Then change the hand positions and continue for a further 1–2 min.

   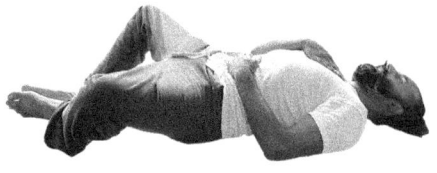

   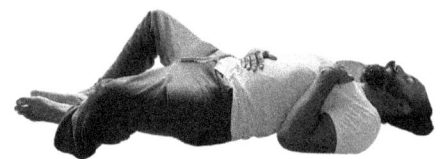

YOGA FOR FREEDOM

6. **Piston kicks.** Lie on the back; engage core abdominal muscles, piston kick the legs by drawing one knee in towards the chest as the opposite leg extends straight around 30–40 cm above the ground. Breathe powerfully in rhythm to the motion. Move quickly so that the breath becomes almost like a breath of fire. 2–3 min.

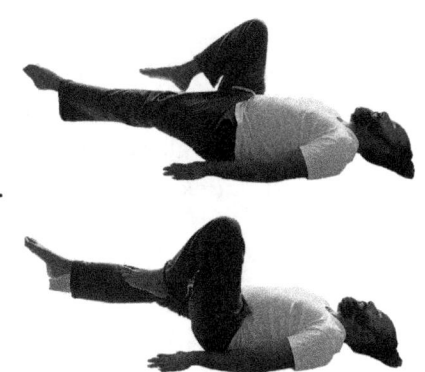

7. **Forward bends to plough.** Lie on the back, extend straight arms along the ground directly behind the head. Inhale, sit up and extend arms forward, hands towards toes. Exhale, return back to the original position and then lift the legs up straight through 90 degrees towards a plough position. Inhaling, release the legs back to the ground. Continue this sequence. 2 min.

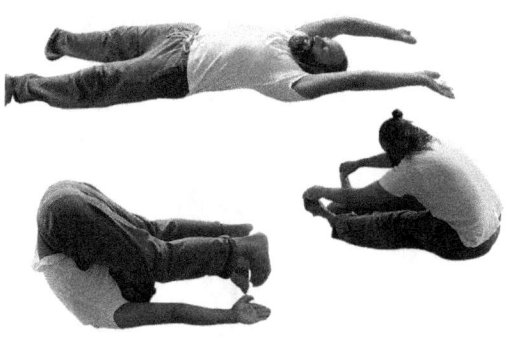

8. **Back platform with breath of fire.** Sit upright with the legs extended straight out along the ground with your arms by your side. Next, raise the body up into a platform shape. Make sure wrists are in line with shoulders, also make sure that ankles are not collapsing outwards. Continue with breath of fire for 1–3 min.

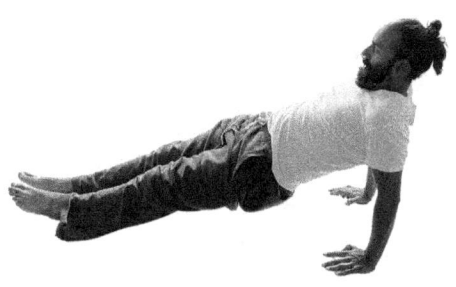

9. **Bow pose with breath of fire.** Lie on your front and grab hold of the ankles, lift the chest and aim to come up high while keeping the knees narrow. Do with breath of fire, 1–3 min.

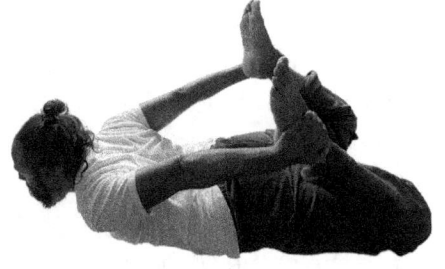

10. **Crow pose with breath of fire.** Come into a crow squat, feet flat on the ground and squatting as close to ground as your body will allow. Extend the arms forward – interlace the fingers with index finger extended. Breath of fire. 2–3 min.

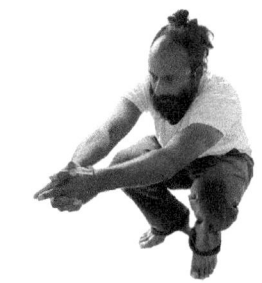

11. **Kundalini lotus.** Seated, hold on to big toes with first two fingers. Balance on pelvis, with spine lifted at the base and extend the legs up and out, forming a wide V shape with your legs. Begin breath of fire for 2–3 min. (Get the legs as straight as possible without compromising elevation of the lower spine.)

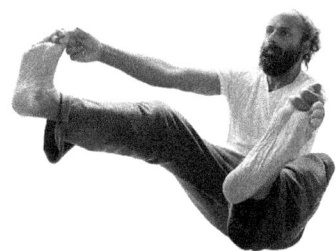

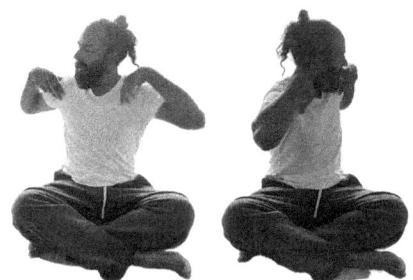

12. **Spinal twist.** In easy pose, place the hands on the shoulders, inhale as you twist left, exhale as you twist right. 2–3 min.

13. **Triple Har.** In easy pose, fingertips touching navel, chant 'Har'. 1–2 min. Move fingertips to chest, chant 'Har'. 1–2 min. Finally, touch fingertips above head, and chant for 1–2 min.

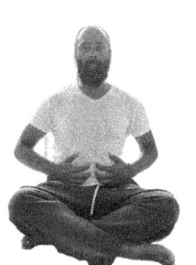 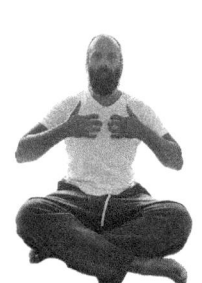 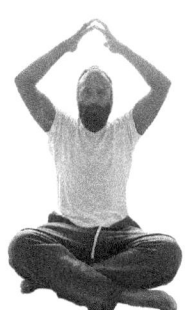

> **Har** is a powerful mantra; my experience of it is that it activates our inner connection power. One could call it raw power. Yet Har relates to the divine emanation of power. One could say the manifestation energy required to bring the blueprint into form. The mantra Har can be chanted more profoundly by striking the roof of the mouth with the tip of the tongue and at the same moment dynamically drawing the navel into the spine with each utterance of Har.

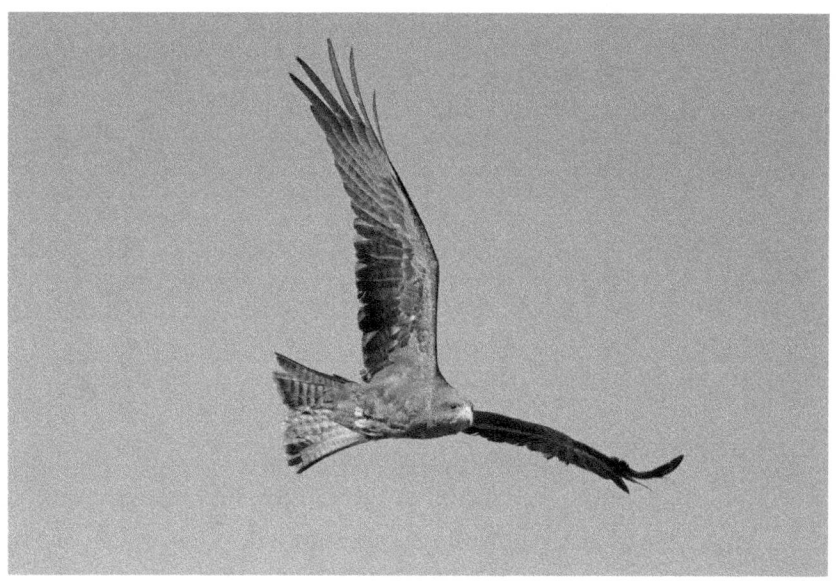

Blue sky

Sometimes we need to drop all concepts, all that we know and allow ourselves the respite of nothingness.

Where we shut down all our inner programmes and allow.

We welcome a blank canvas.

No striving to do and no objective to hit. Just the pure potential.

Give this some space and time before opening to activity again.

Free from conditioning, call on inspiration to fill your canvas, hold back on the habit of concept or conditioning to shape the future.

Let inspiration have its day, behold the power of your own inner wisdom to fly in the blue sky of potential.

The 'true' blueprint takes form in such ways.

1. **Standing arm swings.** From standing, swing arms in backward circles, moving freely and swiftly. Inhale as arms come up, exhale as they come down. 2–3 min.

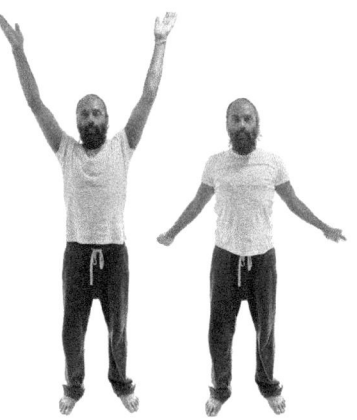

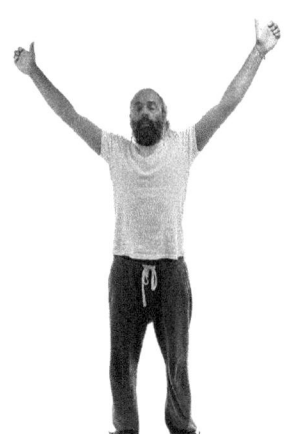

2. **Standing 60-degree arms.** Stand with arms at 60 degrees, fingers drawn into the top part of the palms, thumbs extended, breath of fire. 2 min.

3. **Standing bowing yoga mudra.** Stand with feet slightly wider than hips. Fingers interlaced behind the back, exhale, bow forward as arms rise up. Inhale and torso rises back up and arms relax down. 2–3 min.

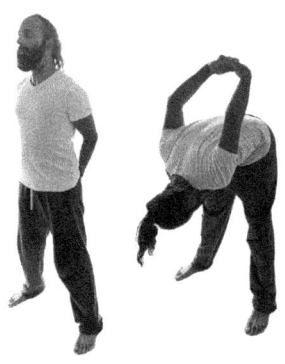

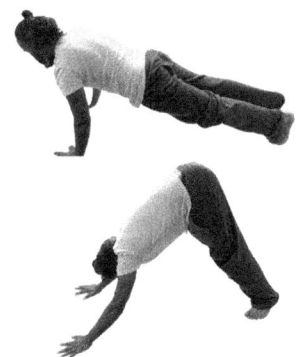

4. **Front platform to downward dog.** From front platform (plank), inhale into downward dog. Exhale back into front platform. Continue for 2–3 min.

5. **Rocking bow.** Lie on your front and grab hold of the ankles, lift the chest and aim to come up high while keeping the knees narrow. Breathe long and deep, allow the breath to take you into a natural rocking motion. 1–3 min.

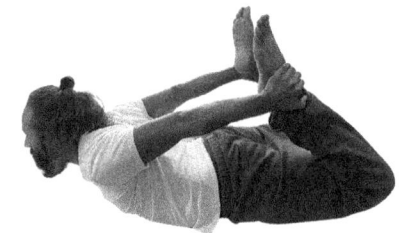

6. **Stretch pose.** Lie on the back, engage the core muscles of the stomach, bringing the lower back into the ground. Lift the legs up 15–30 cm, and the head up the same height and gaze at the toes, the arms come up to the sides. Have a feeling of lengthening (stretching) the body in this position. 1-3 min with breath of fire.

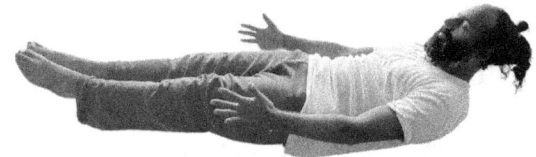

7. **Knees in jump.** Hug the knees to the chest, nose between the knees – attempt to jump the body off the ground while in this position. 1–2 min.

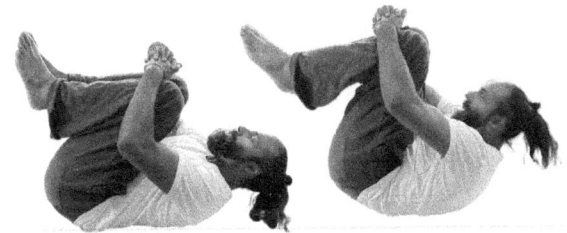

8. **Wide knees navel pump.** Keep knees wide, sit back on heels, support yourself with your hands behind you keep the torso straight at an angle of around 60 degrees. Inhale – exhale and hold the breath out. Pump the navel for as long as you can with the breath held out. When you can't hold the breath out any longer inhale – exhale, hold the breath out and repeat the process. 3 min. To finish, inhale and hold.

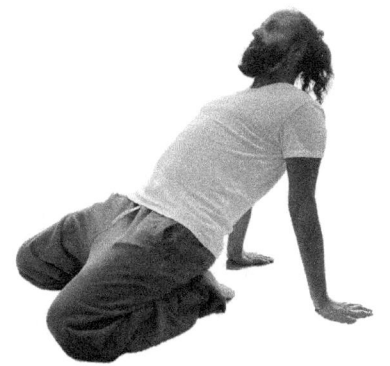

9. **Heavenly corkscrew.** In a kneeling position, extend the arms up above head, palms together. Rotate torso. As if 'corkscrewing' to the heavens. Move with devotion. 1–2 min then change direction, continue 1–2 min.

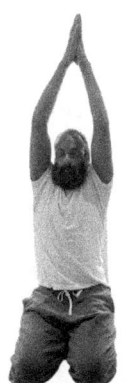
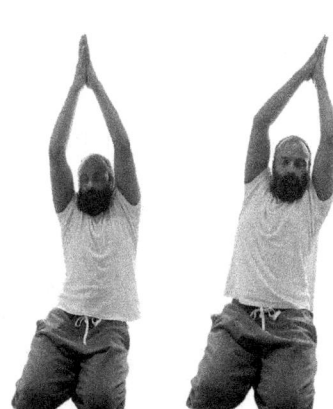

10. **Halo arms O-breath.** In easy pose, interlace the fingers above the head. Form an O-shaped mouth with a powerful breath, breathe via the mouth. 2–5 min.

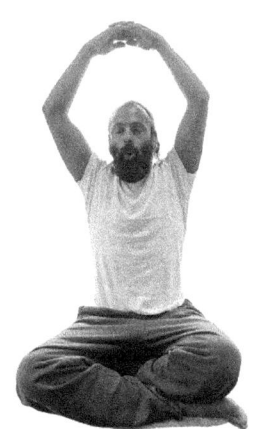

11. **Chant 'Lakshmi mantra'.** Sitting in easy pose, chant 'Om Shri Mahalakshmi Namah'*. 3–11 min.

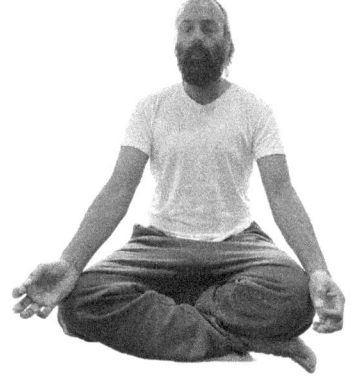

> Om Shri Mahalakshmi Namah. Lakshmi is the goddess of wealth and prosperity, beauty and fertility. Basically, all the aspects that we would seek to engender in our everyday lives. The mantra gives a sense of support in the daily tribulations and trials of life, evoking the goddess energy brings a sense of exceptional motherly support to our lives.

🎧 Music suggestion: Lakshmi mantra by Jaya Lakshmi and Ananda

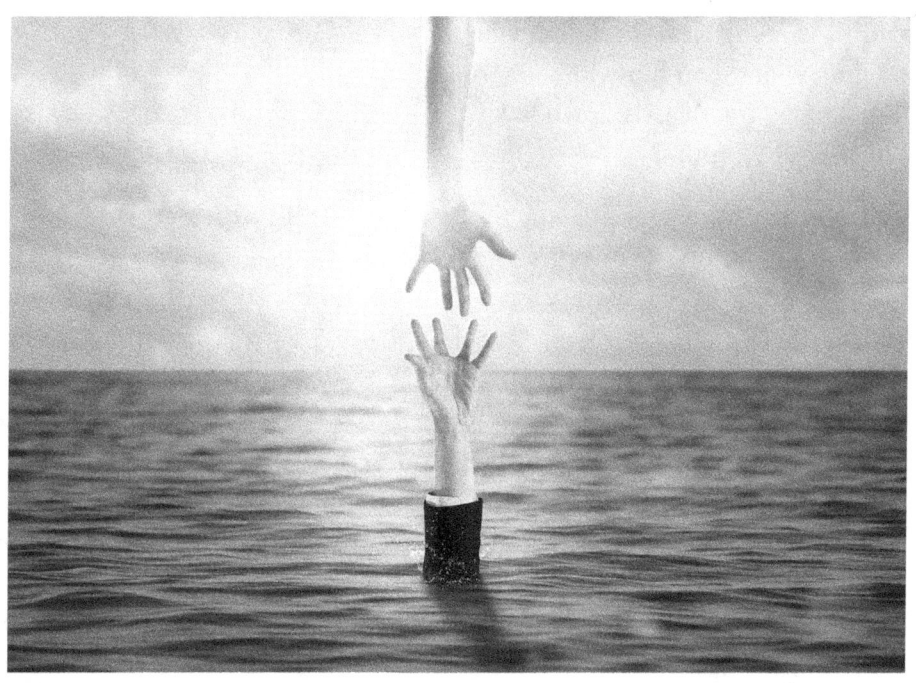

Giving it to source

Pride is a force that is most delicate. Pride in some circles is applauded: he is proud of his children; they are a proud nation; she takes pride in her work. Yet it is an aspect of ego, albeit with a veneer or gold plating.

Pride is a function of maya, and as such, is best relinquished or redirected. Anything that is tethered to ego shall be limited and will never give you what life really is asking of you. Pride points to you as the doer and this is the route of all malaise.

You must give your glory – your pride – to divine. Only then can divine carry your suffering. Through the concept of sin, you feel you must suffer, but this is not the case if you open to the divine hand.

1. **Standing torso twist.** Standing with feet a little wider than hip-width, arms at right angles, inhale twist torso to left, exhale to right. 2 min.

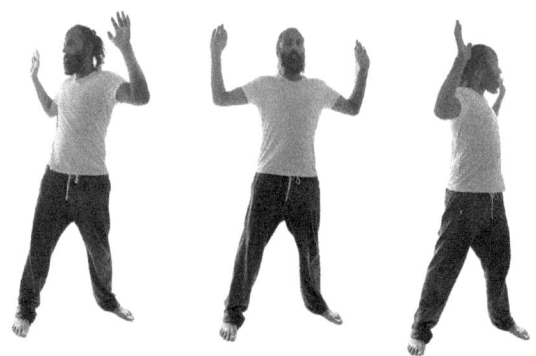

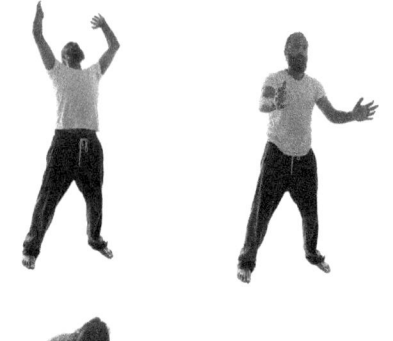

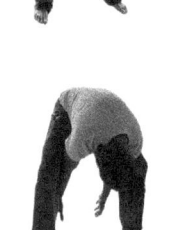

2. **Hold the sun swing.** Stand with the feet slightly wider than the hips, reach up tall holding your sun, with a very slight back bend as you inhale, then exhale, fold forward from the waist, allowing the lower back to be free. Bend your knees slightly as you fold forward – this is a very relaxed free movement. 2–3 min.

3. **Standing eagle pose**. Bend the right knee slightly then bring the left knee over the right knee and place the left foot behind the calf of the right leg. Then place the right elbow on top of the left elbow crease and place the palms of the hands together. Press the palms together to open the shoulders and sit a little deeper through the right knee. 1–2 min. Change sides and repeat for 1–2 min.

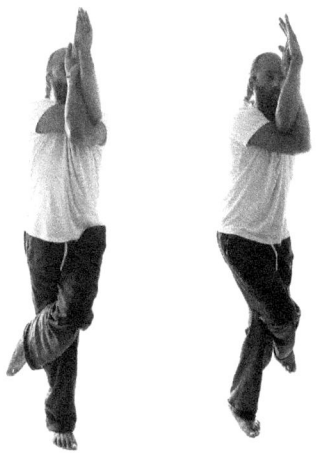

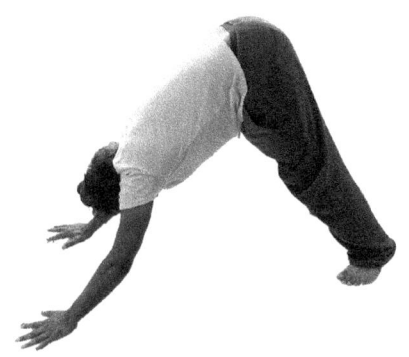

4. **Downward dog**. Come into downward dog. On all fours, with knees beneath hips and hands beneath shoulders, lift the buttocks off the ground coming on to the toes. Straighten the legs creating a triangular shape with the body (or shape of a dog stretching). 2–3 min.

5. **Chest raises**. Lie on front, inhale for count of five as you lift the chest off the ground, stretching the arms back behind you. Hold for a count of five, then exhale and lower to ground across a count of five. 1–2 min.

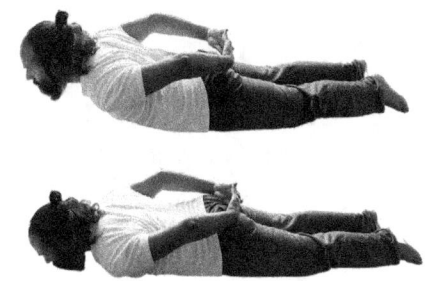

6. **On knees spinal twist**. Sitting back on the heels and on the knees, place the hands on the shoulders, inhale as you twist left, exhale as you twist right. Continue, 2–3 min.

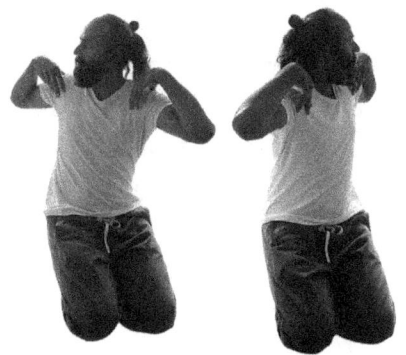

7. **On back steady hold**. Lie on back, raise up arms, shoulder-width apart, fingers to ceiling with palms facing. Legs raised 90 degrees. Chant 'Om Mani Padme Hum'. 2–5 min.

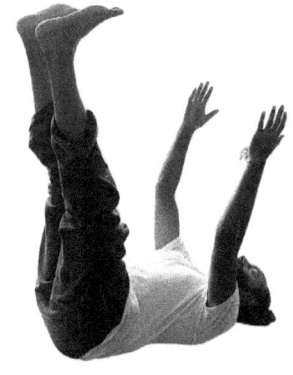

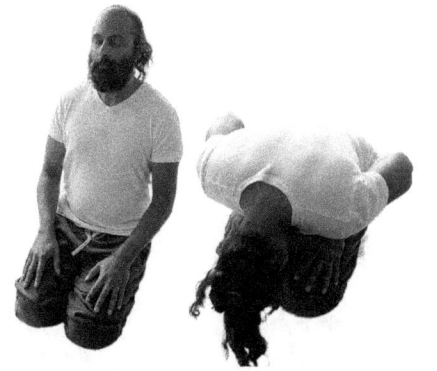

8. **Bowing with Om Mani Padme Hum***. Come to a kneeling position, bow the head to the ground in time to one recitation of Om Mani Padme Hum and return to the upright position, on one recitation. Continue to bow up and down in rhythm to the mantra. 2–5 min.

9. **Hands on chest chant***. Seated in easy pose, hands on chest, chant 'Om Mani Padme Hum'. Continue 2–5 min.

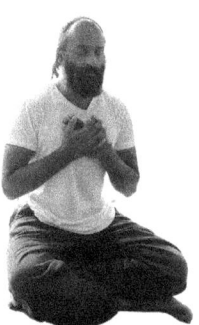

Om Mani Padme Hum is a delightful mantra. It has energetic resonance and devotional verve while being powerfully harmonious. It points towards the lotus flower that resides in the heart. The heart is said to be the seat of the soul. The effect is a reminder to ourselves of our own true home.

🎧   Music suggestion: Om Mani Padme Hum by Veet Vichara and Premanjali

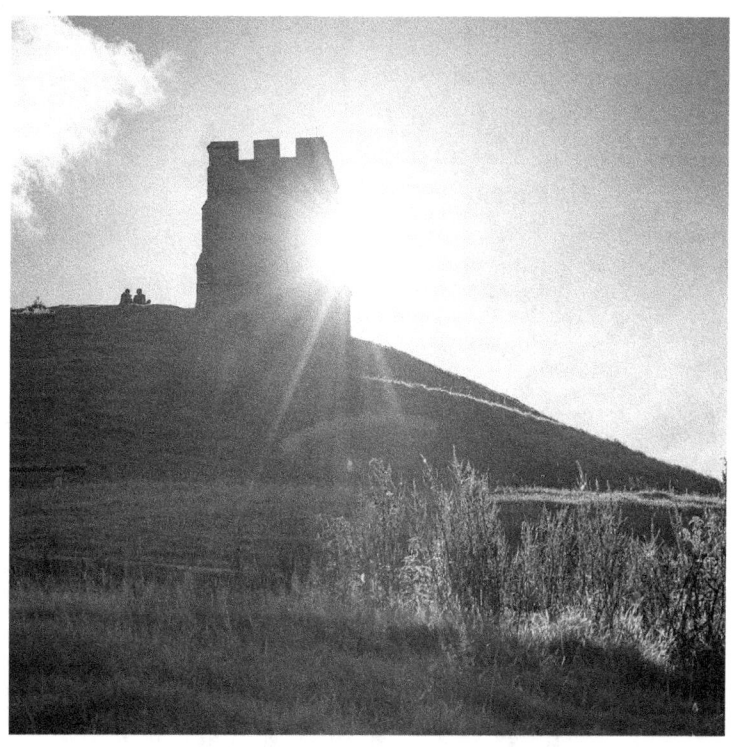

Developing steadiness

Our security and peace are not discovered in the concepts and creations of the external world. Or indeed in the more intimate sphere of our mind.

We can very literally create castles in the sky, yet even the most powerful of citadels throughout the history of time have fallen.

Peace remains elusive in such places. We must realise that true peace lies beneath the illusion of maya. Peace is not something that is only available to the rich and powerful; it is something that all may reach should they ignite a purity of discovery.

Cultivate the bridge between manipura and anahata to discover the foundation for peace. In this direct experience we will be free.

1. **Dancing spine.** Come to all fours, then begin to move the spine from side to side; initiate the movement through the hips. 1.5 min. Next, add an up-and-down motion to the existing lateral movement; effectively 'dancing the spine'. 1.5 min.

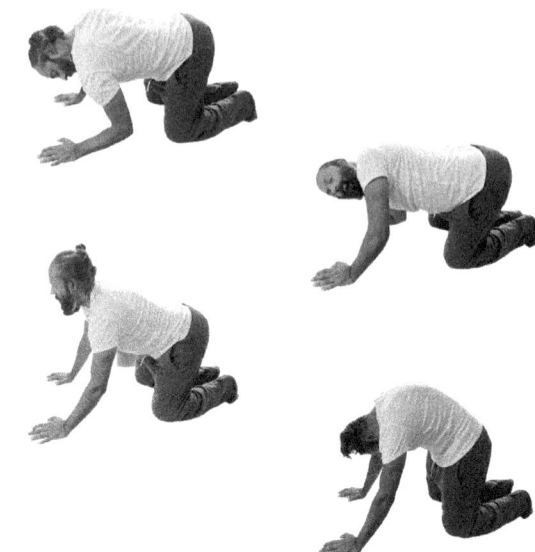

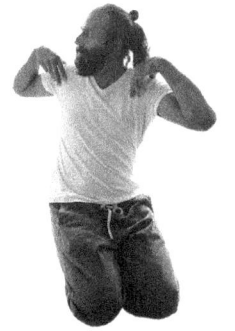 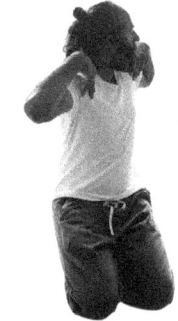

2. **On knees spinal twist.** Sitting back on the heels and on the knees, place the hands on the shoulders, inhale as you twist left, exhale as you twist right. 2–3 min.

3. **Stretch pose.** Lie on the back, engage the core muscles of the stomach, bringing the lower back into the ground. Lift the legs up 15–30 cm, and the head up the same height and gaze at the toes, the arms come up to the sides. Feel like you are lengthening (stretching) the body in this position. 3 min with breath of fire.

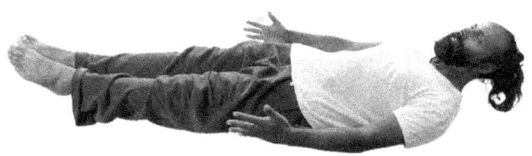

4. **Half wheel breath of fire.** Lie on the back, knees up, soles of feet on ground. Press through the feet to lift the pelvis off the ground. Hold elevated position and begin breath of fire. 2–3 min.

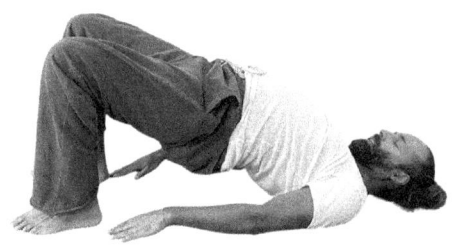

5. **Piston kicks.** Lie on your back, engage the core stomach muscles, left knee comes into chest, arms by the side (hands beneath lower back if required) right leg extended straight and hovering 15–30 cm off the ground (this is inhale position), exhale and switch legs like a piston, right leg comes in, left leg reaches out. Move with powerful breath 2–3 min.

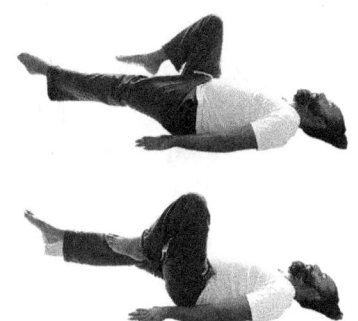

6. **Bear grip with breath of fire.** Sit in easy pose with bear grip, the right palm faces inwards about 15–20 cm away from chest and clasps the fingers of the left hand, which faces away from the body. The elbows are out to the side. Face and shoulders relaxed, keep a gentle tension in the grip and keep the arms parallel to the ground. Breath of fire. 3 min.

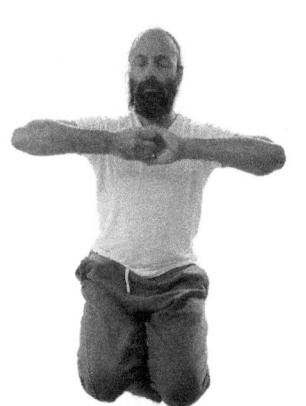

7. **Extended arms prayer.** Sit in easy pose, cup the hands and extend the arms straight in front of you keeping them parallel to the ground. Inhale in 10 strokes through the nose. Exhale in 10 strokes through the nose. 2–11 min.

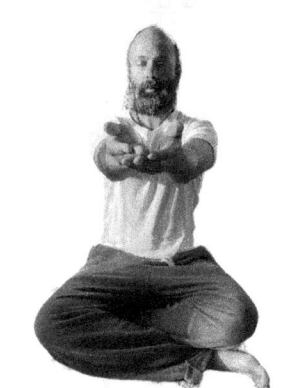

8. **Downward dog held.** Come into downward dog. On all fours, knees beneath hips, hands beneath shoulders, lift the buttocks off the ground coming on to the toes. Straighten the legs creating a triangular shape of the body (or shape of a dog stretching). 1–3 min.

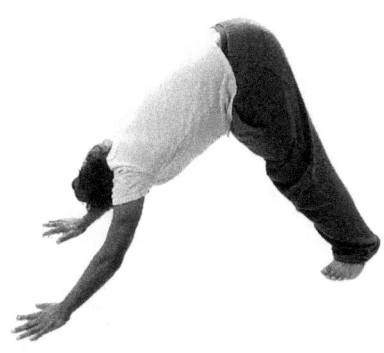

9. **Cobra up and down.** Lie on front, inhale through the nose, push up into a cobra as you exhale, through the mouth over extended tongue (lion breath). Inhale through the nose as you come back down. Continue the movement and breath. 3–7 min.

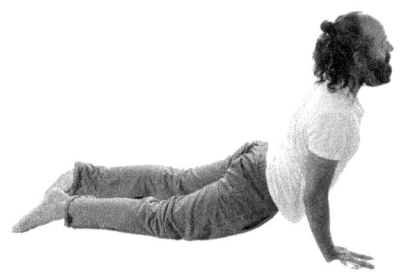

10. **Ganapati mantra – *Om Gam Ganapati Namah.**
    Chant the mantra – 5–11 min.

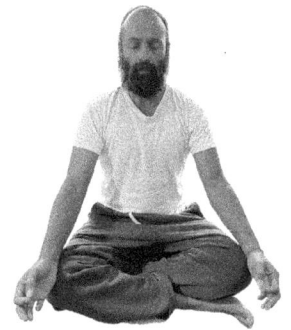

Om Gam Ganapati Namah. Ganesha the deity evokes so much fondness within the Hindu religion (and in modern times beyond …). Classically known as the remover of obstacles, but in reality he is so much more. He is the first to evoke with any new projects and offers straightforward ballast in life challenges and endeavours.

🎧 Music suggestion: Om Gum Ganapatayei Namaha by Deva Premal

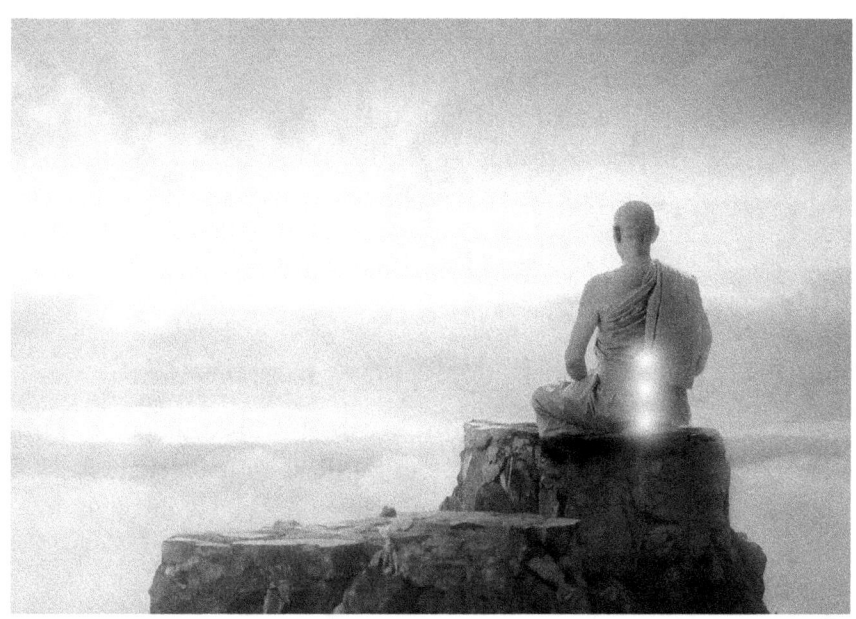

Return to the essence

As we emerge into the freshness of a new season – especially spring – we are imbued with a newness, a sense of expressing ourselves authentically.

This shows itself naturally in our external world; we may be drawn to freshen up our wardrobe or to spring clean the whole house. These are very natural and welcomed behaviours, yet if one does not clean at a deeper level, they may turn out to be merely sticking plasters across wounds not fully healed.

What I talk of here is an exploration of our first three chakras. They are fundamental to transformation as they anchor our sense of self-concept and manifest identity.

They are the functional energy centres by which we engage with the world around us. If we make the effort to cleanse and clear, we shall create the foundation for a sustained evolutionary expression of self.

Essence alludes to a refinement or distillation to find the magical attribute that conveys the signature frequency; to do this we must include everything and hide nothing. The primary 3 chakras contain the richest of raw materials by which we can turn lead into gold.

1. **On back buttock kicks.** Lie on your back, bring legs up to 90 degrees then kick your buttocks with alternate heels (if heels don't reach get as close as). Exhale through the nose as each heel strikes the buttocks. 1–3 min.

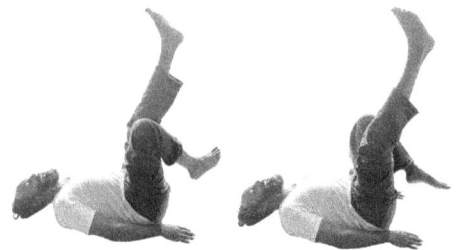

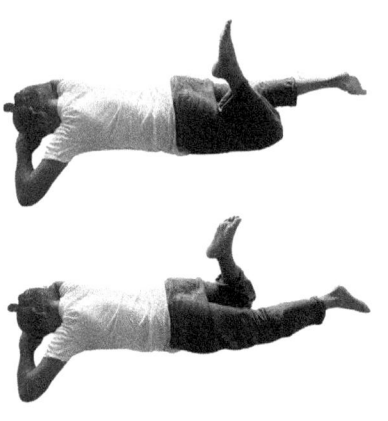

2. **On front buttock kicks.** Lie on your front then begin to kick your buttocks with alternate heels (if heels don't reach get as close as). Exhale through nose as each heel strikes the buttock. 1–2 min.

3. **On knees Sufi swirl.** Sit on heels. Place hands on the knees, sitting bones on the floor. Next, begin to make large circles with the spine and as you do so inhale as you rotate the body forward and exhale as you rotate the body backwards. Move like a swirling Sufi. 2–3 min.

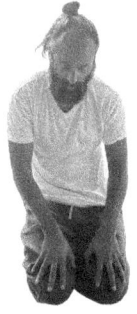 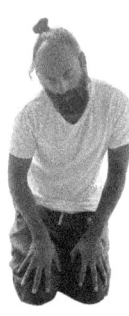

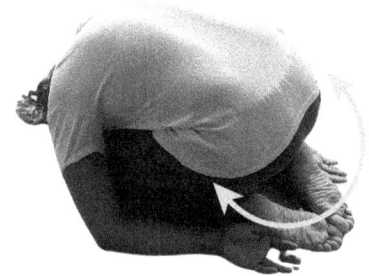

4. **Baby pose dragon tail rock.** Sit back on the heels in child's pose, move the buttocks in a U shape. The movement is deep and visceral moving into the hip joint. Imagine you are moving a big heavy tail! 3 min.

5. **Just sit.** Sit and be; meditate. 1–2 min.

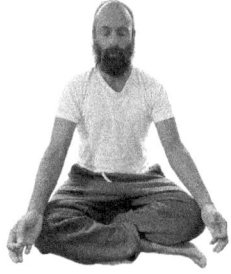

6. **Torso hold.** Extend the legs straight out along the ground, arms are straight and parallel to the ground, palms face each other, shoulders back, chest open, lean torso back 60 degrees. Hold position and begin breath of fire. 1–3 min.

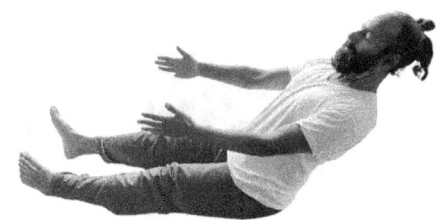

7. **Frogs.** Come into a squatting position, heels together, toes out, hands together and fingertips on the ground. Inhale as you straighten the legs, allow torso neck and head to drop forward. Exhale, return to the original position. 1–2 min.

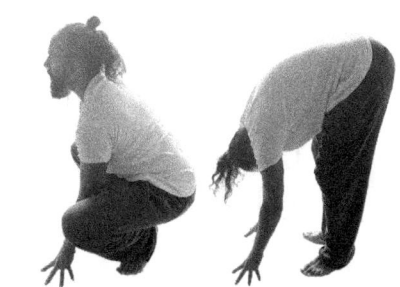

8. **Spinal flex.** Sit in easy pose. Hold on to the shins, begin to flex the spine. Inhale forward, exhale back. 2–3 min.

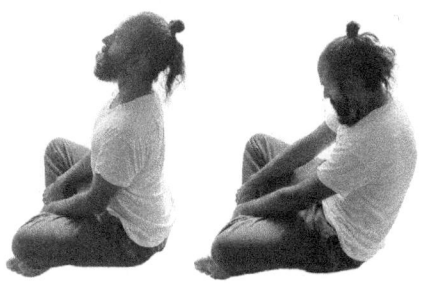

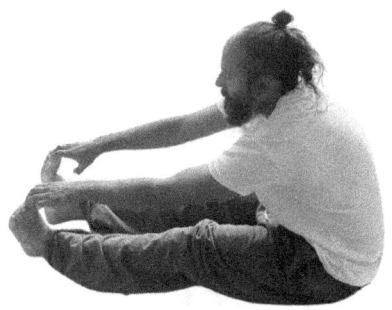

9. **Life nerve.** Sit with the legs out straight, reach forward and grab the toes or shins, begin breath of fire. 2–3 min.

10. **Activated Hari Naam mantra.** Sit on heels in kneeling position. Raise arms above palms together, apply the neck lock. Chant 6 x 'Har' and 1 x 'Hari Naam' powerfully from the navel area, the breath happens naturally between each utterance. 3–7 min.

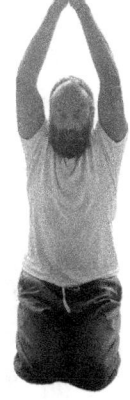

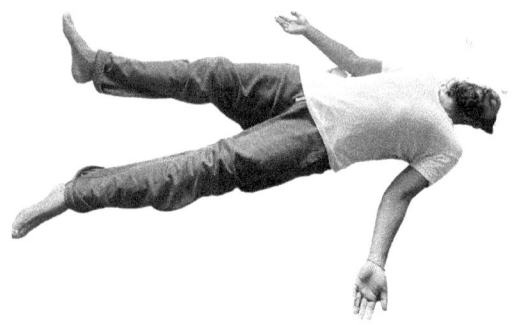

11. **Lie on back.** 1–2 min.

12. **Dance on ground.** Lie on your back and dance your body on the ground, moving arms, hips and feet, be rhythmic and dynamic. 1–2 min.

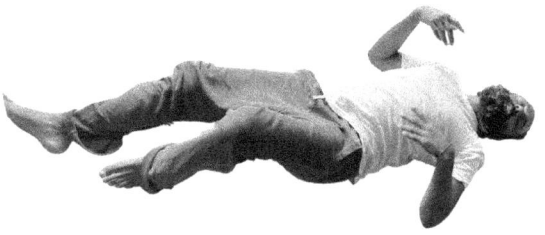

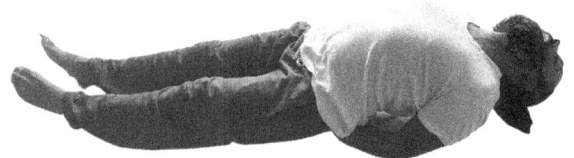

13. **Fish pose.** Lie on the back, arms reach under the body, hands beneath buttocks / upper thighs. Raise torso up on to the forearms (arms bearing all the weight), allow the chest to open and release the head back to the floor. Ensure the arms are strong and stable – breathe long and deep. 30–60 seconds.

14. **Rhythmic cat stretches.** Laying on your back, extend the arms out to the sides, palms facing up. Knees up, soles of the feet on ground. Exhaling, drop the knees to the left and turn your head towards your right shoulder. Inhale as you bring the knees back to centre, exhale as the knees drop towards the right, turning your head towards your left shoulder. Keep going with this movement paying attention to harmonising the movement of lower and upper body. Stay relaxed but speed up once the rhythm of movement has been obtained. 3 min.

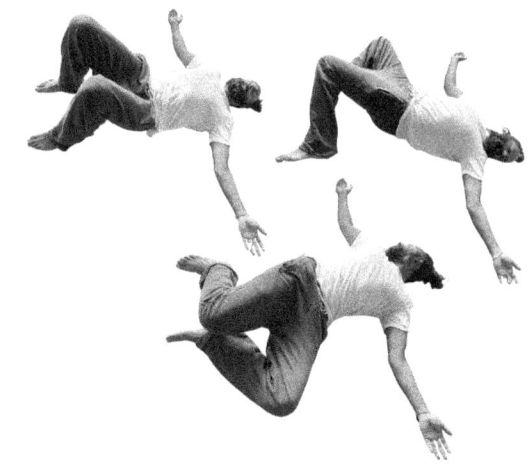

15. **Celestial Green Tara mantra.** Chant the *'Green Tara mantra' with the following movements.

Om Tare – Palms face forward by shoulders.
Tu Tare – Palms turn in 90 degrees, fingers point up elbows by ribcage, palms and forearms aligned.
Ture – Arms extend straight up at an angle of 60 degrees.
Svaha – The hands come to centre of the chest, right on top of left.

Repeat for 3–11 min.

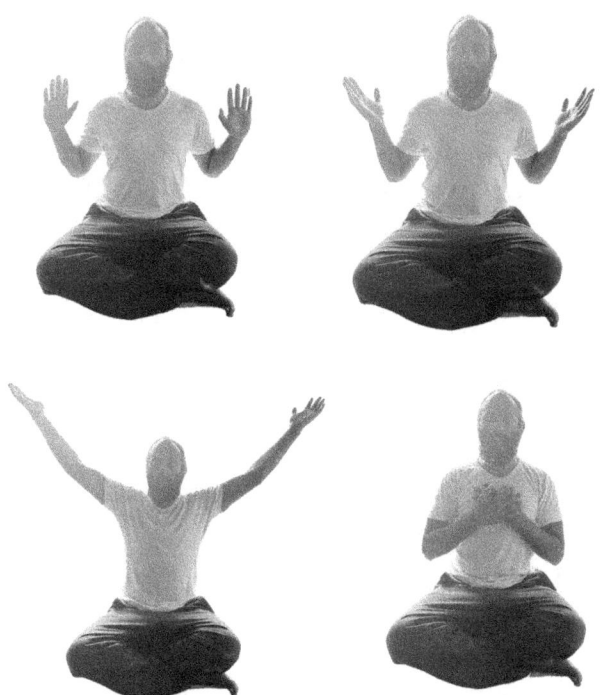

Green Tara has a special place in my heart. Her presence has been pivotal during transitions in my life, her boundless compassion is very magical. The mantra is wonderfully devotional, the movements that I decided to add felt a nice way to step into the devotional energy.

🎧   Music suggestion: Om Tare Tuttare by Deva Premal

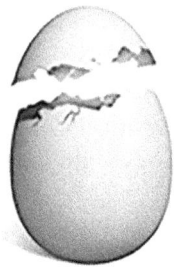

Crack open the shell

The shell is something that we can all relate to; it has such a wide range of related metaphors.

The shell of a snail may evoke a sense of home from home–a kind of caravan of liveability.

The tortoise when threatened retracts all vulnerable parts. To leave the would-be attacker a virtual tank casing to penetrate.

Seashells are often taken home as small treasure, as a keepsake from a holiday or may comprise the materials of a striking piece of coastal art.

Then perhaps we move to the most common shell of all, eggshells.

These seemingly dormant entities are full of the potency for creation – waiting to be activated before coming into life.

I once witnessed some swans that were guarding a mighty set of eggs. There were many interested parties to these eggs, many onlookers keen to see progress. The expectation was magical; would they witness a birth?

Then on one afternoon, all that remained were the remnants of broken shells scattered to the ground. In their place lay younglings ready for a new cycle of life.

In this sense a shell offers a polarity, its job is to contain and protect, yet at some point it needs to relinquish its duty and surrender to its fate.

The wisdom for us is to know when the time is right to come out of our shell?

1. **On knees spinal flex.** Sit in kneeling position. Hands on lap, inhale flex spine forward, exhale flex backwards. Eyes closed focussed on brow. 2–3 min.

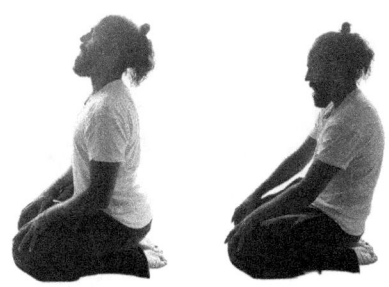

2. **Seated row.** Sit with the legs out straight, inhale and reach forward through the arms and torso keep legs straight, exhale and come back, lean back slightly, draw the hands in towards the armpits – chest opens. Inhale, reach forward once again–continue with this rowing-like action for 2–4 min.

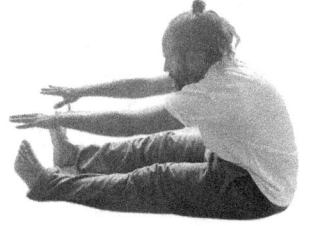

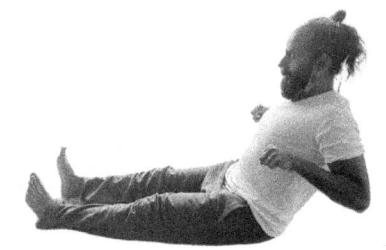

3. **Alternate leg lifts.** Lie on the back and begin alternate leg lifts. Inhale, left leg up, exhale, bring it down, inhale, right leg up, exhale, down. 2–5 min.

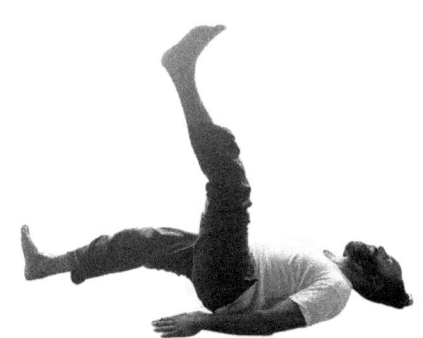

4. **Stretch pose.** Lie on the back, engage the core muscles of the stomach while bringing the lower back into the ground. Lift the legs up 15–30 cm, and the head up the same height and gaze at the toes, the arms come up the sides. Have a feeling of lengthening (stretching) the body in this position. 3 min with breath of fire.

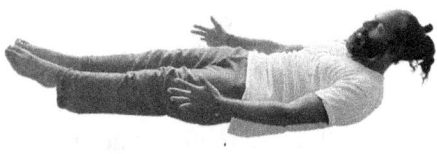

5. **Full/half wheel.** Lie on the back, knees up, soles of feet on ground. Press through the feet to lift the pelvis off the ground. Hold this elevated position and begin breath of fire. 2–3 min.

6. **Walk the dog.** Come into downward dog: on all fours, knees beneath hips and hands beneath shoulders, lift the buttocks off the ground coming on to the toes. Straighten the legs creating a triangular shape of the body (or shape of a dog stretching). Hold for 1 min. Then start to walk the legs up and down, inhale up, exhale down. 2 min.

7. **Cobra with breath of fire.** Lie flat on your front, bringing the hands beneath the shoulders, keeping the legs nice and relaxed, slightly engage the core muscles of the lower abdomen. Inhale and press up into a cobra position. Hold this position with breath of fire for 2–3 min. (Come into sphinx pose if preferable, forearms on ground, elbows under shoulders.)

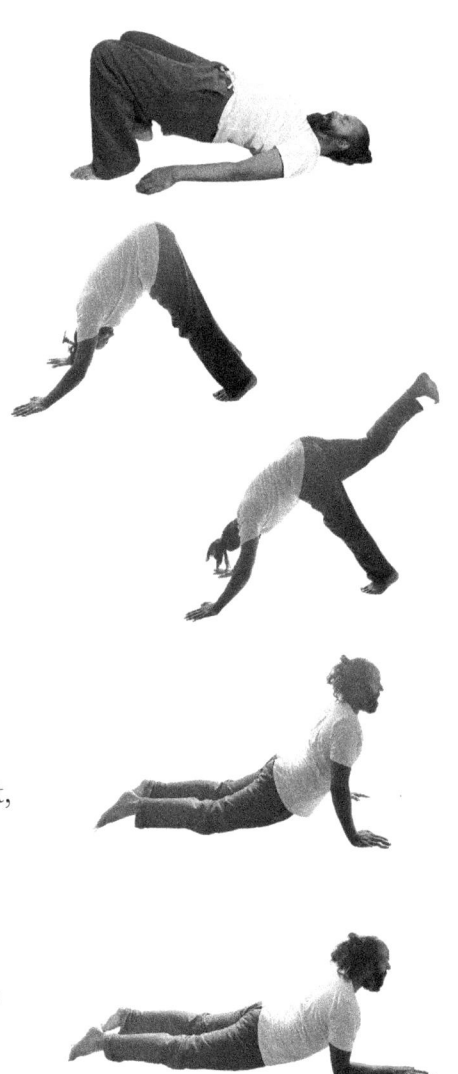

8. **Frogs.** Come into a squatting position, heels together toes out, hands together and fingertips on the ground. Inhale as you straighten the legs, allow torso neck and head to drop forward. Exhale, return to the original position. 1–2 min.

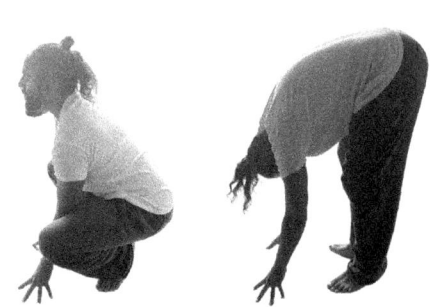

9. **A pranayama sequence.** Easy pose, block right nostril with thumb of right hand. Inhale through left nostril slowly until lungs are full. With little finger of right-hand block off left nostril and exhale through right nostril till empty. Continue like this for 2–3 min. Finish on the exhale and rest for 10–30 seconds. Then block left nostril with thumb of left hand, inhale through right nostril slowly until lungs are full. With little finger of left-hand block off right nostril and exhale through left nostril until empty. Eyes closed focusing on brow. Continue for 2–3 min.

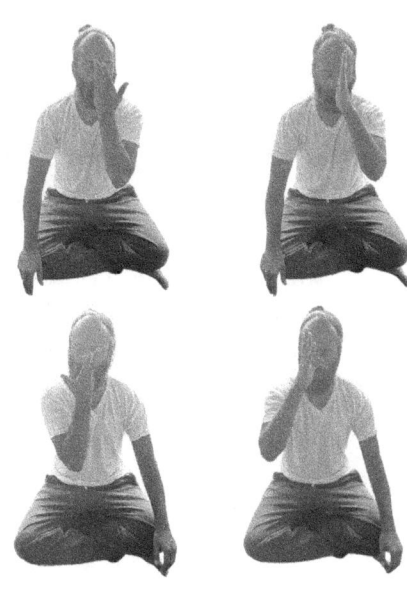

10. **On knees punch.** Sit back on the heels, bring the hands into fists and begin to punch with alternating arms. Exhale on impact (full reach of each arm – without locking the elbow). 3–5 min.

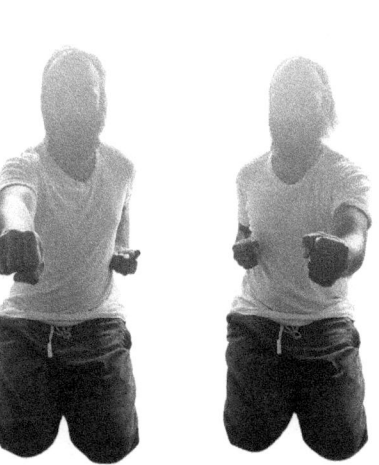

11. **On knees arm pumps.** Sit in a kneeling position – fingers interlaced with each other and arms extended straight out ahead. Inhale forcefully and equally forcefully bring the arms up, exhale forcefully and bring the hands down. Continue this dynamic movement of the arms. 2–3 min.

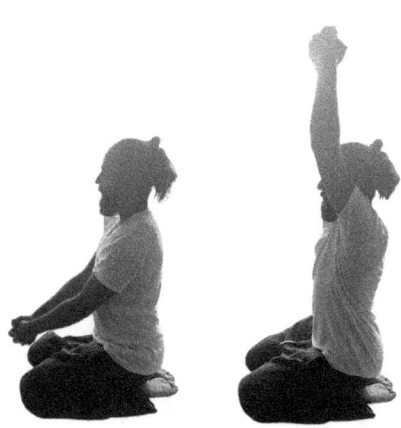

12. **Dynamic shoulder rolls.** Easy pose, hands in relaxed fists by the shoulders, move in a dynamic fashion by rolling your shoulders back, brining your shoulder blades together. Repeat this action quickly and dynamically, the breath is through the nose and in rhythm with the motion. 3–5 min.

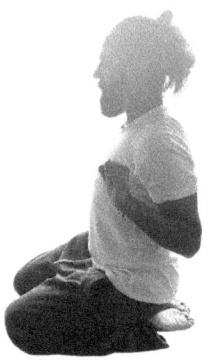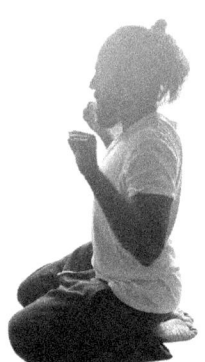

13. **Savasana**. 5–11 min.

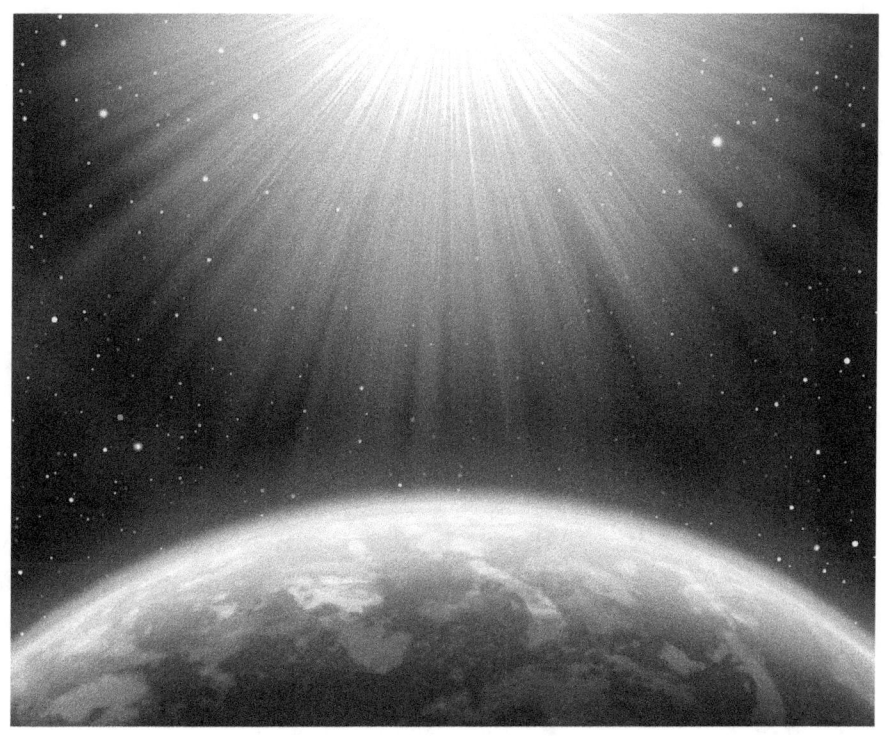

Heaven to earth

Our soul purpose can sometimes feel ephemeral or 'fantastical'. Belonging more in the realm of fairy tales than embodied reality. Our soul purpose emits in the higher vibrational field of the upper chakras principally sahasrara (7th chakra). The one thousand-petalled lotus. It exists at our crown … conveniently out of sight, we are left guessing what it's really all about?

We try to reach up and grab it but at best we retrieve snippets of information that only add to the mysteriousness of it all. After a while the unreachability of spiritual life becomes the game. It becomes the drama of a whole pseudo-culture. We make a whole business of pretending or almost living a spiritual life, it's a very easy thing to do – most clever.

Yet at some point if we are lucky enough it becomes unbearable, we cannot deal with the fake – so we go hard and deep and we become real. We do the heavy lifting and we decide to embody the life of our highest calling; it is a seismic shift as you don the robes of your incarnation you become the pathfinder. You bring heaven to earth.

1. **Standing prance.** March/prance on the spot staying on the toes as best you can, move with swagger and rhythm. 1–3 min.

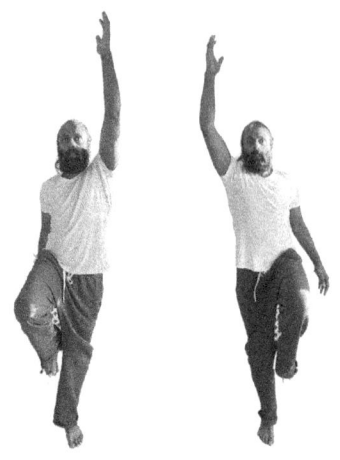

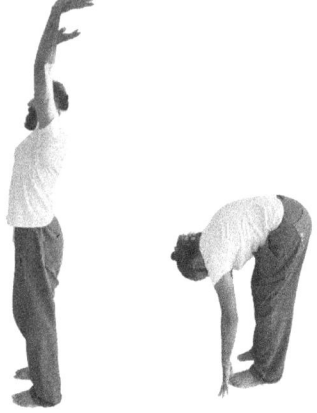

2. **Miracle bends in time with Kali/Durga mantra** (if you can) *. Standing straight, feet hip-width apart, arms up, palms face ceiling, slight back bend. Slowly exhale and bend towards the ground for one verse. Inhale slowly as you rise back up to the original position with the next verse. Continue and move with awareness. 3 min.

3. **Tepee fingers with breath of fire.** Easy pose, hands 30 cm above head, fingers spread and tips of fingers from each hand touch each other. Breath of fire. 2–3 min.

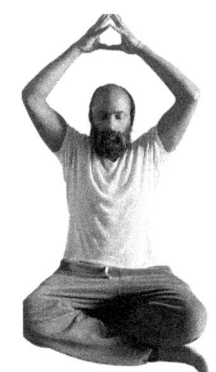

4. **See-saw arms (third eye).** Easy pose arms straight and shoulder-width apart level with the eyebrows, move the arms up and down moving no lower than the chest and no higher than approximately 10 cm above the crown. Move the hands in rhythm to a breath of fire. 2–3 min.

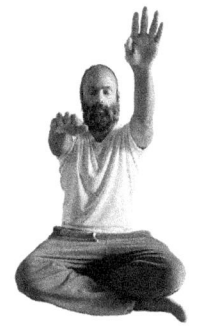 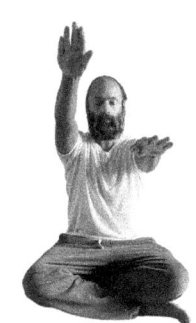

5. **Easy pose neck turns.** Sit in easy pose, turn head left inhale, exhale turn head to right. 1–3 min.

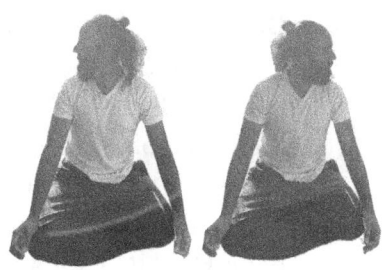

6. **Walking on hands and feet.** Hands and feet on the floor knees may bend. Begin walking on all fours, on the spot, opposite arms and leg are raised each time. Move rhythmically and fluidly. 2–3 min.

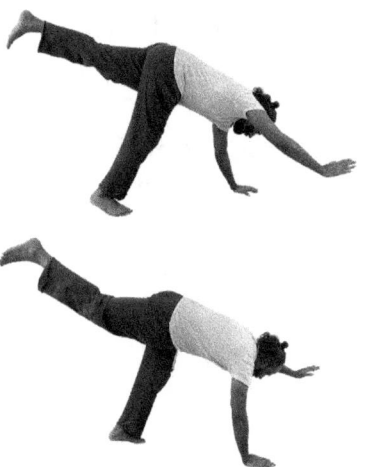

7. **Plank and side plank.** Come into plank, front platform position. Then come into a side plank, keeping the left arm in alignment with the shoulder move to a side-on position with the left arm with stacked feet holding the body weight. Right arm is extended upward – hold with breath of fire for 20–30 seconds. Return to front platform then change sides. Right arm bearing the weight – 20–30 seconds with breath of fire.

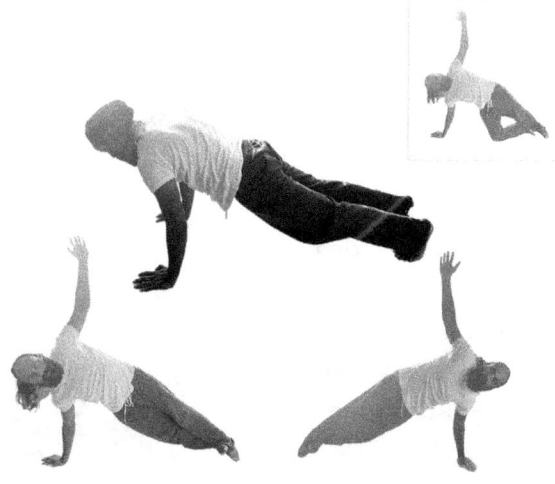

8. **Bow pose up and down (with 'Om So Hum').** Lie flat on your front, reach back with the hands and grab hold of the ankles. Inhale across the recitation of the mantra *'Om So Hum', push back with the feet and ankles into the hands, allowing the chest and upper thighs to rise off the floor. Hold here for a recitation of the mantra 'Om So Hum'. Exhale for the recitation of the mantra 'Om So Hum' as you lower yourself back to the ground. Keep repeating this process, each time allowing the body to open and release a little more, remain very aware of the breath and body. 2–5 min.

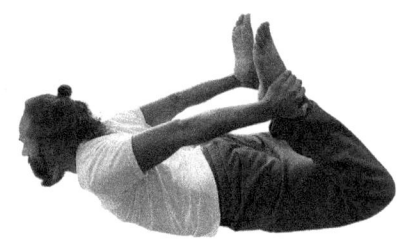

9. **Cat cow.** Come on to all fours, begin to flex the spine. Inhale as the spine arches downward and the head rises (cow). Exhale as the spine arches upward and the head releases down (cat). Move smoothly, gradually increasing the speed as the body opens. 2–3 min.

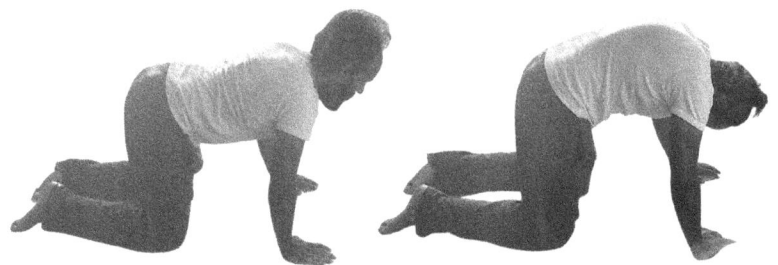

10. **Downward dog and rest on thigh.** Come into a downward dog hold for 1 min then raise up the right leg high and behind – swing it through bringing the right leg into kneeling position. Lower the torso over the right thigh, extend the left leg straight and behind, then bring arms down either side of the body, rest here 2 min. Inhale and bring yourself back to downward dog, rest here 1 min, then repeat the same process this time with the left leg … rest on the left thigh 2 min once again. Finish inhale and bring yourself back to easy pose.

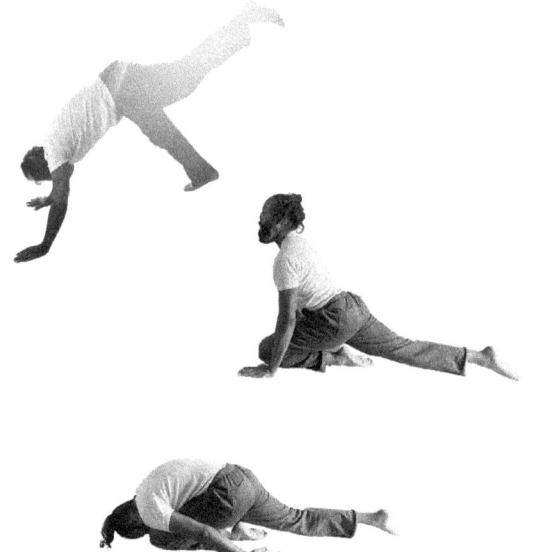

YOGA FOR FREEDOM

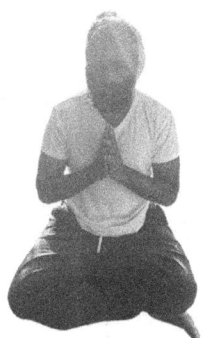

11. **Inhale breath hold 5 times (breath retention).** Hold each breath for 1 min. If that is not possible start with a shorter time, e.g. 30 seconds, and build up.

12. **Heaven to earth with *Om Gan Ganapati.** Come into horse pose, legs wide, knees bent. Raise the arms high up, chant 'Om Gan Ganapati Ye Namah', then bow down straighten legs and recite once again. Come back up into the original position – keep repeating this cycle. 3–5 min.

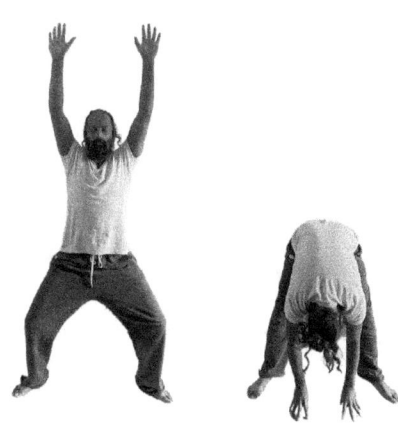

13. **Just sit and be.** 1–2 min.

14. **Shoulder stand/plough.** Come on to the back and bring your knees up, soles of feet on the ground. From this position lift your knees towards your head and support your back with your hands, keeping your elbows and upper arms on the ground so as to support your torso. Walk the hands as far up the back as you find comfortable then extend the legs up towards the sky. Lifting the legs out of the hip sockets, toes point to the ceiling. Keeping the neck open and free. (2–3 min)

15. From shoulder stand – lower into plough by allowing the legs to drop down over your head bringing the toes to ground and legs straight. (1–2 min)

16. Relax 8–15 min

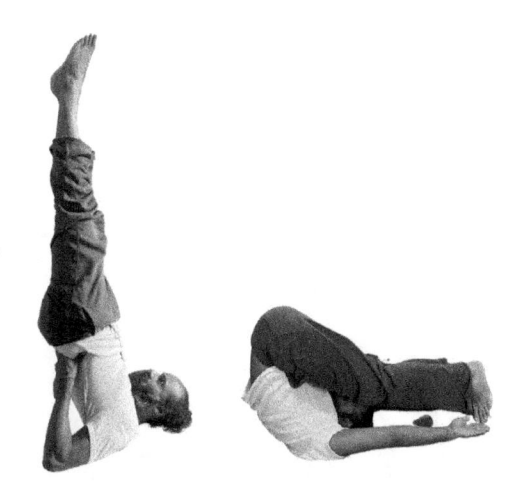

> Kali and Durga are two powerful goddesses from Hindu mythology. Chanting this mantra evokes their inspiration and protection (should you have need).
>
> Om So Hum is very much a mantra of the heart. It in someways is a deep dive into the very centre of one's essence. It asks us to remember our true divine nature and its abode, which lies within and without.
>
> We mentioned Ganesha in another kriyā, but here we open to his powerful grounded nature, which provides the perfect platform for celestial growth.

🎧 Music suggestion: Kali Durge by Mantra Tribe

🎧 Music suggestion: Om So Hum by Luca´Spirit

🎧 Music suggestion: Om Gum Ganapatayei Namaha by Deva Premal

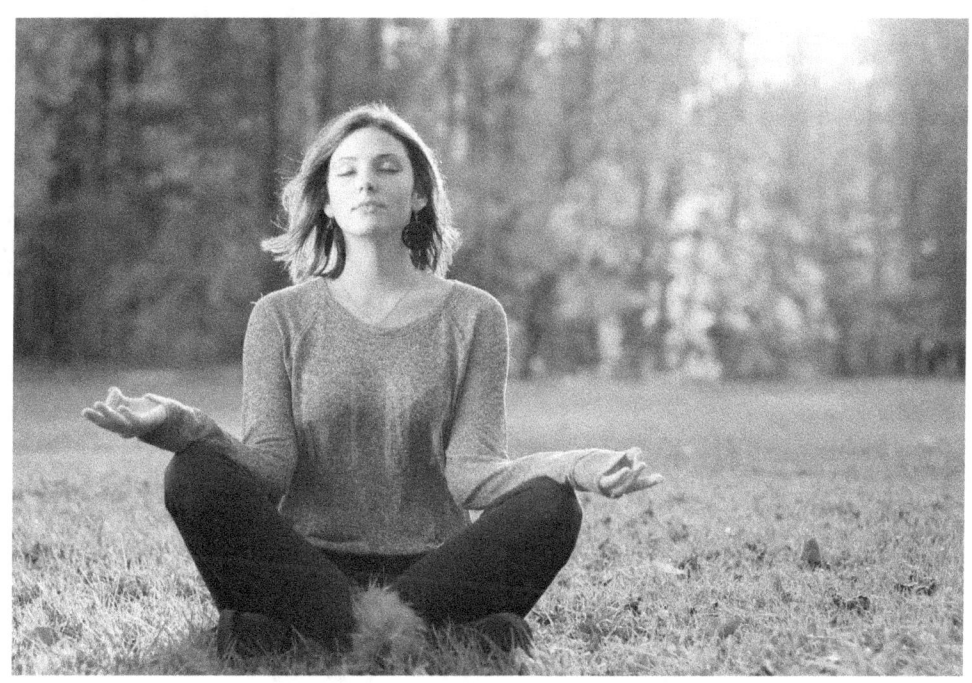

Stillness is the new norm

How we have come to disempower stillness. It seems to have dropped down the pecking order of human endeavour. Ironically lost within the smorgasbord of spiritually inclined practices. In the celebration of practice prowess, we forgot the treasure itself. The mind is fiendish in that regard. We need mind to coordinate our inspiration, but we must not promote mind to the creative director's chair. If we do stillness will be forgotten.

Stillness lies beyond the remit of statue artists; it delves instead into the inner dimension of activity. Our inner world manifests our outer world, stillness is sought within the chambers of our corrupted mind. We seek the key to unlock the room in which it is caged.

When freed stillness reveals its might, like an elixir of love it has the capacity to flood all of mind, allowing it to serve once again the one.

1. **Standing dance/shake.** Standing hip-width apart, arms relaxed by your side, begin to quickly flick the legs out, keeping the legs quite straight, at the same time shaking the lower arms wrists and hands. Keep the movement relaxed fluid and dynamic. Continue for 2–3 min.

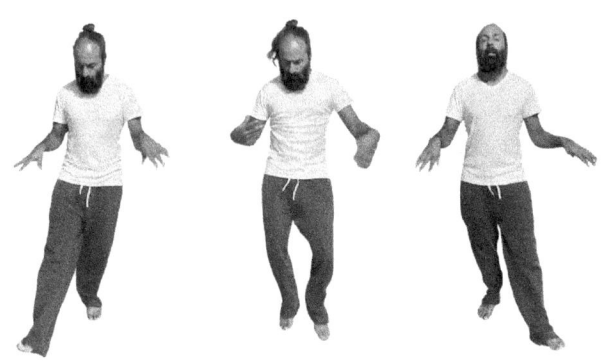

2. **Standing torso rotations**. Standing hip-width apart, hands on hips, rotate the torso in large circles keeping the legs and hips as stationary as possible. Change direction of rotation a few times during the duration of exercise. Continue 3–4 min.

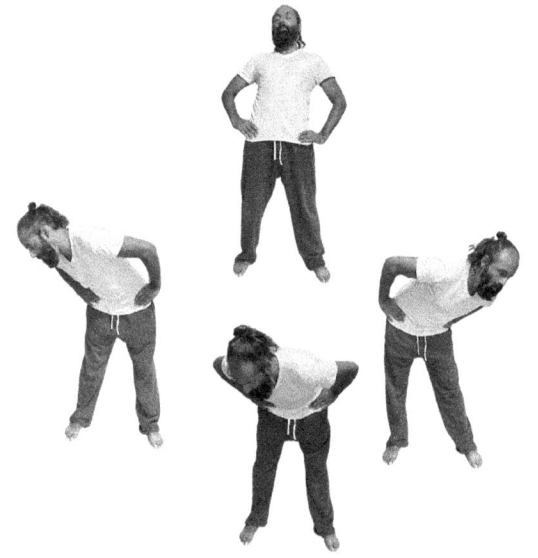

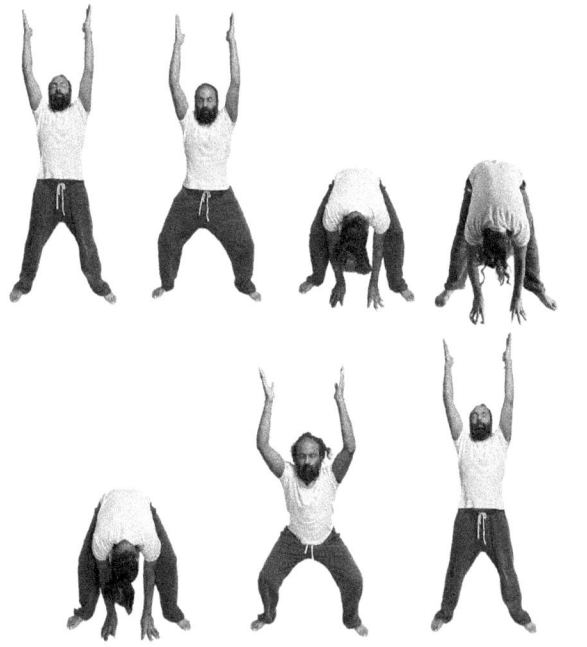

3. **Wide leg squat and fold**. Standing legs wide, arms straight up above the head, squat down then bend forward from the waist bringing the hands to the floor. Then straighten the legs with the hands on the ground. Return to the squatting position, arms return above the head, finally straighten the legs, and return to the original position. Repeat the sequence, 3 min.

4. **Kidney diagonals.** Rise up on to knees, right leg out to the side, left hand on left hip, right arm reaches out diagonally to the left, forming a straight line with torso and leg. Continue with long deep breathing for 30–60 sec. Repeat on the opposite side.

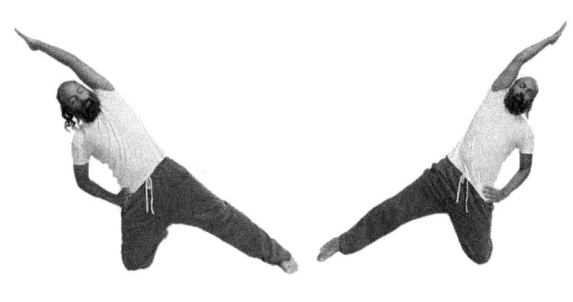

5. **Kidney raises.** Sit back on heels, palms together on the ground. Elbows just in front of the knees. Staying very relaxed in the lower back and tailbone area, draw your torso up and above the forearms on the inhale. Exhale and return to the original position. Continue 3 min.

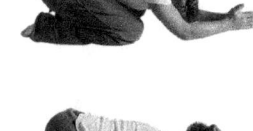

6. **Nabhi flower.** Lie on back, hug knees into chest, inhale as you extend the legs out straight at an angle of 60 degrees, at the same time the arms go wide out to the floor, continue this movement dynamically and devotionally. 5–7 min.

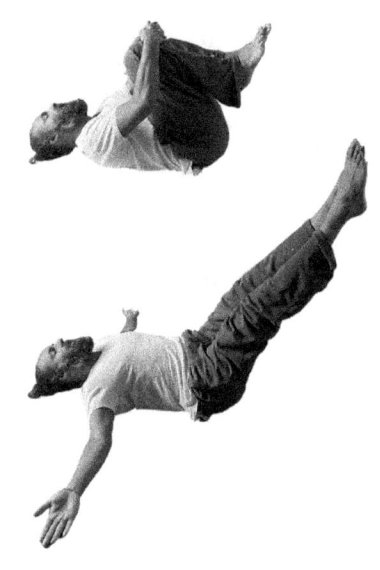

7. **Held half wheel.** Lie on back, knees up soles of feet on ground. Press through the feet to lift the pelvis off the ground. Hold elevated position and begin breath of fire. Continue for 2–3 min.

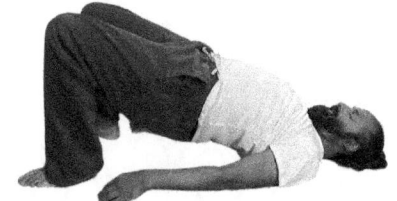

8. **Pranayama 8-stroke breath.** Sit in easy pose, inhale in 8 strokes through the nose. Exhale in 8 strokes through the nose. Continue for 3–5 min.

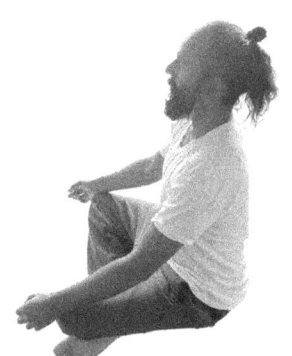

9. **Frog twists.** Squat heels together, toes pointing away at around 45 degrees. Fingertips outstretched on ground just in front of the feet. Look up like a frog. Inhale, straighten legs, keep left hand on the ground and twist to the right, extend the right arm up towards the sky. Return the right hand to the ground, exhale as you return to original position. Repeat with the opposite side. 2–3 min (20–30 repetitions).

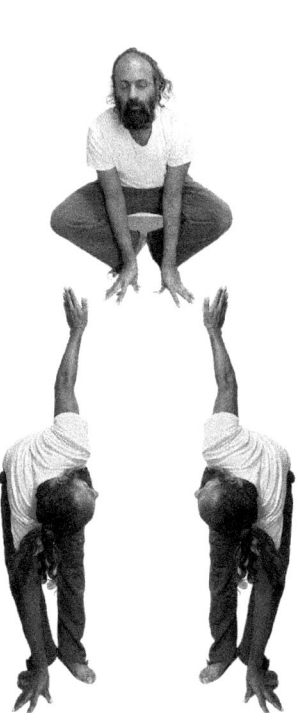

10. **Savasana** (10–15 min)

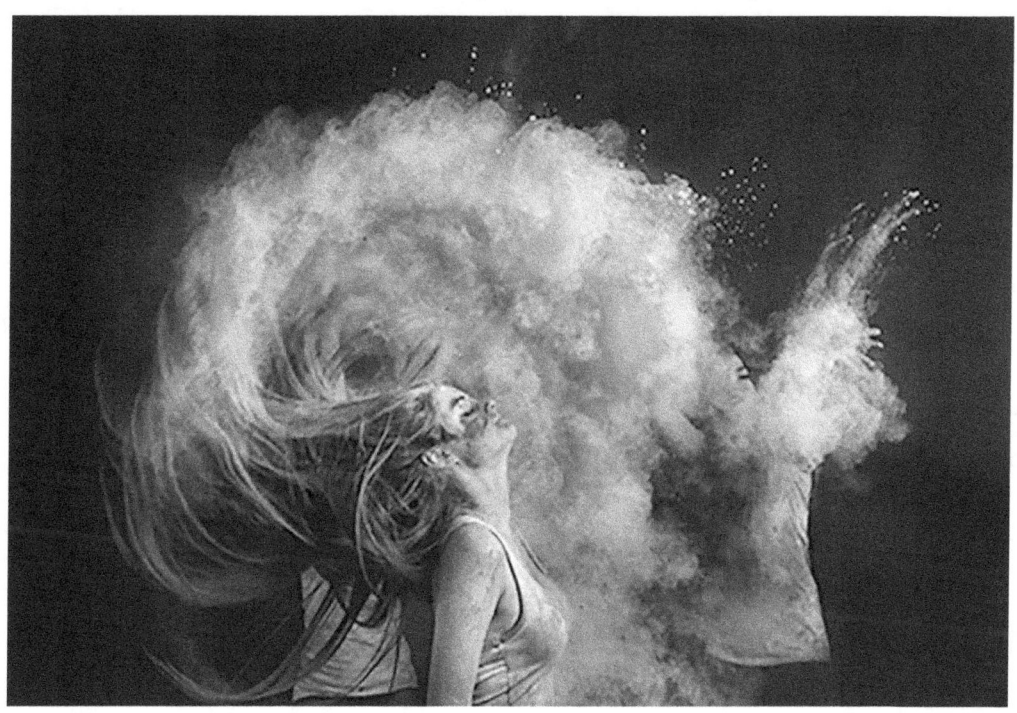

Essence of expression

We can sometimes skirt around an issue, some may call it a merry dance, or simply building up to the punchline.

You may love preamble, seeing it as a necessary or useful warm-up to the main event or NOT, but what we probably all can agree upon is that we value the essence of our engagements.

The essence is akin to the treasure of a holy grail, or the lock & key to meaningful being.

We may have been conditioned to not touch our essence for fear of the consequences. Especially if that which feels primal and authentic to us does not seem to fit into our culture or environment. Yet in the end the essence loves to express itself, when given freedom of expression that essence can be a thing of beauty, one could say it is the very reason for being. Yet if suppressed the essence will reach the surface of the world but shall be corrupted or diminished. A chimera, shadow or echo of its full potential.

1. **Lateral snake spine.** On all fours, move the spine in a lateral fashion, side to side like a snake. Stay relaxed and fluid throughout. 1–2 min.

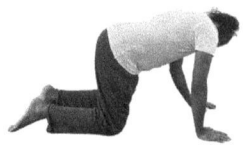
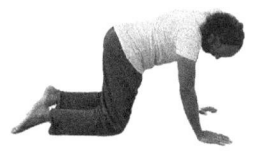

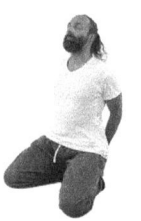
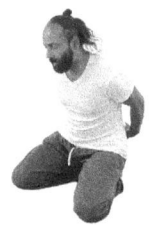

2. **Wide knees yoga mudra.** Sit with wide knees, dance the spine and torso as you bow towards the ground and you lift your arms up behind your body. Do for 3–5 min.

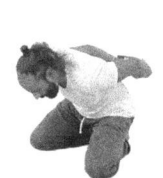
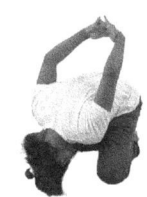

3. **Frogs.** Come into a squatting position on the toes, heels together, hands together and fingertips on the ground. Inhale, straighten the legs, allow torso neck and head to drop forward. Exhale, return to the original position. 1–2 min.

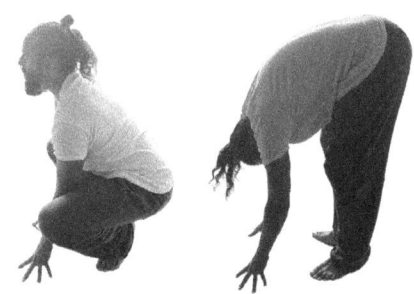

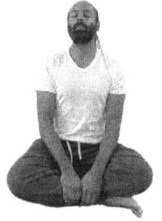
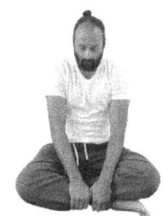

4. **Spinal flex 5s and 7s.** Hold on to shins, flex the spine 5 times across one long inhale. Then flex 5 times across one long exhale. 1–2 min. Then hold knees, continue with flexing movement but this time flexing 7 times across inhale and exhale. 1–2 min.

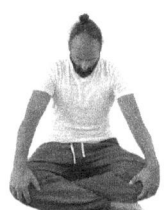
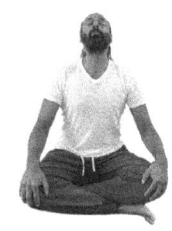

YOGA FOR FREEDOM

5. **Frogs.** Come into a squatting position on the toes, heels together, hands together and fingertips on the ground. Inhale, straighten the legs, allow torso neck and head to drop forward. Exhale, return to the original position. Do for 1–2 min.

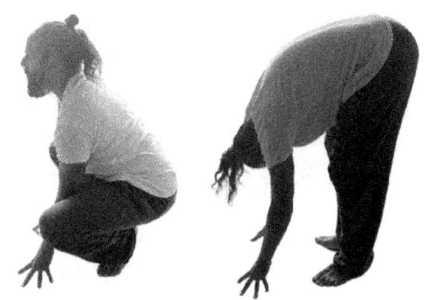

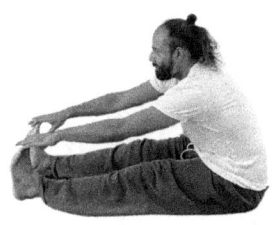

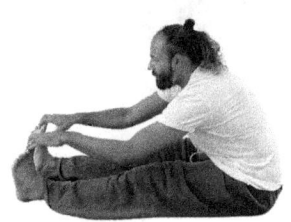

6. **Moving and static forward bend.** Sit and extend legs straight out, hold on to toes (ankles or shins), exhale as you fold forward from the waist. Inhale as you come back up to the original position. 2 min. Inhale, hold the position, exhale – keep the position without moving and begin breath of fire. Continue for 1 min.

7. **On back feet drops.** Lie on your back, exhale and allow your feet to drop out to the sides, inhale and bring the feet back up. Move the feet quickly, keep the legs and body relaxed. 2–3 min.

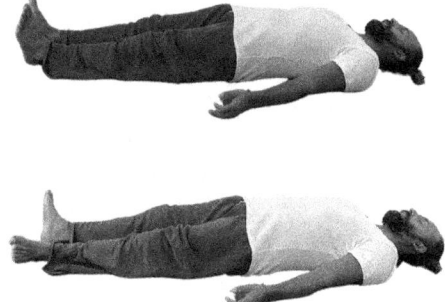

8. **On back side stretch**. Lie on your back and stretch each side of the body alternately, a deep and relaxed stretch through the right side and then the left, keep alternating fluidly 2–3 min.

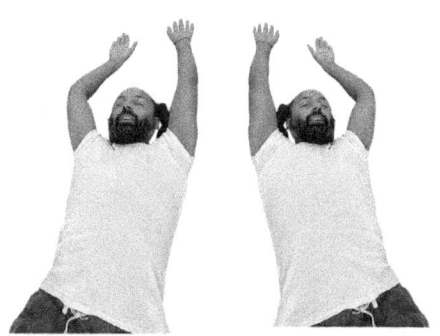

9. **Forward bend to plough.** Lying on your back, engaging your core, reach forward towards your toes, return back to the original position then smoothly continue the movement back into plough, then return back to the original position and on to a forward bend … keep moving like this for 1–2 min.

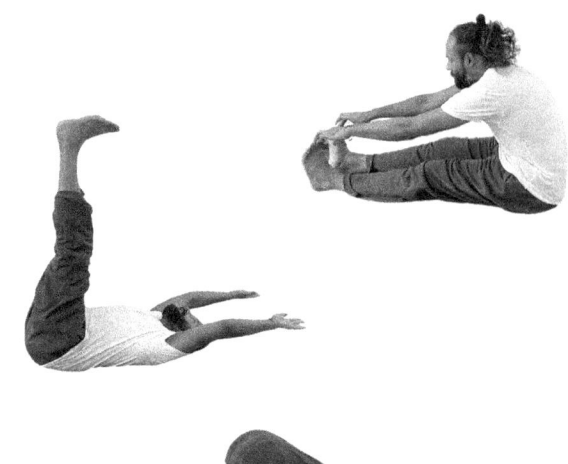

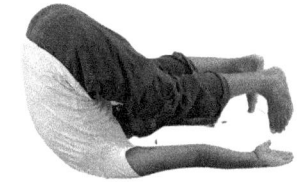

10. **Bear grip swivel.** Sitting back on the heels, left palm faces out, right palm facing, in, interlock the fingers and pull, with enough force to establish a firm grip and enable the forearms to remain parallel to the ground. In this position, 'see-saw' the forearm up and down. 3–5 min.

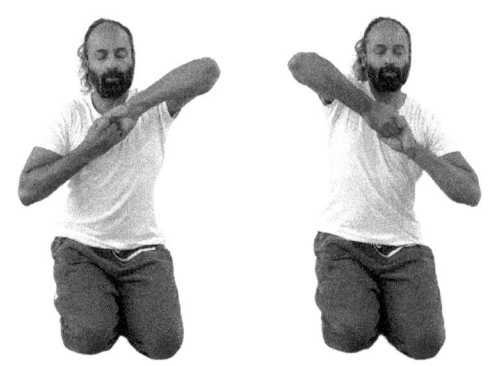

11. **Camel.** Standing on knees, reach back and take the heels with your hands (or lower back if you cannot reach), allow the chest to be open, head drops back (if possible). Breath of fire. 1–3 min.

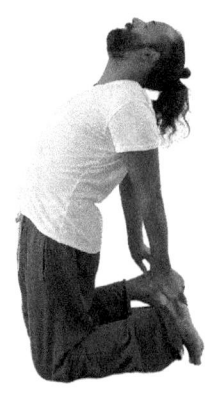

YOGA FOR FREEDOM

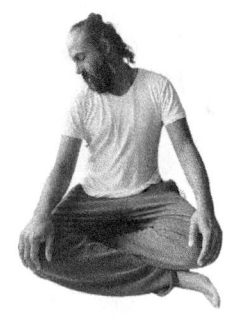 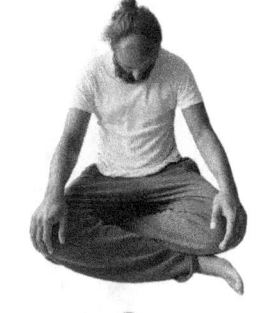

12. **Neck rolls.** Seated, start to roll the head slowly in a circular motion, changing direction a couple of times. 2–3 min.

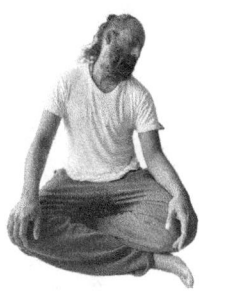 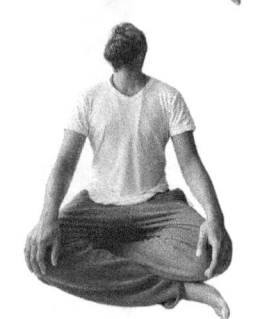

13. **Touch of the heart (with Ahem Prema*).** Seated, touch the centre part of the chest with just the tips of the fingers, touch gently as if 'sensing'. Chant the mantra 'Ahem Prema'. Chant with devotion and feel the sound through the fingertips and in your chest and body. Ahem Prema means 'I am Love'. 5–11 min.

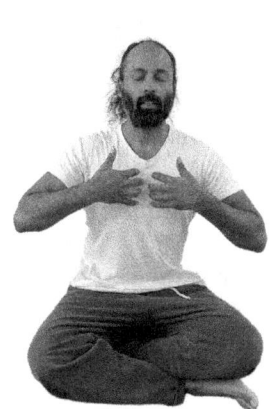

14. **Savasana** – 11 min

🎧   Music suggestion: Ahem Prema by Deva Premal

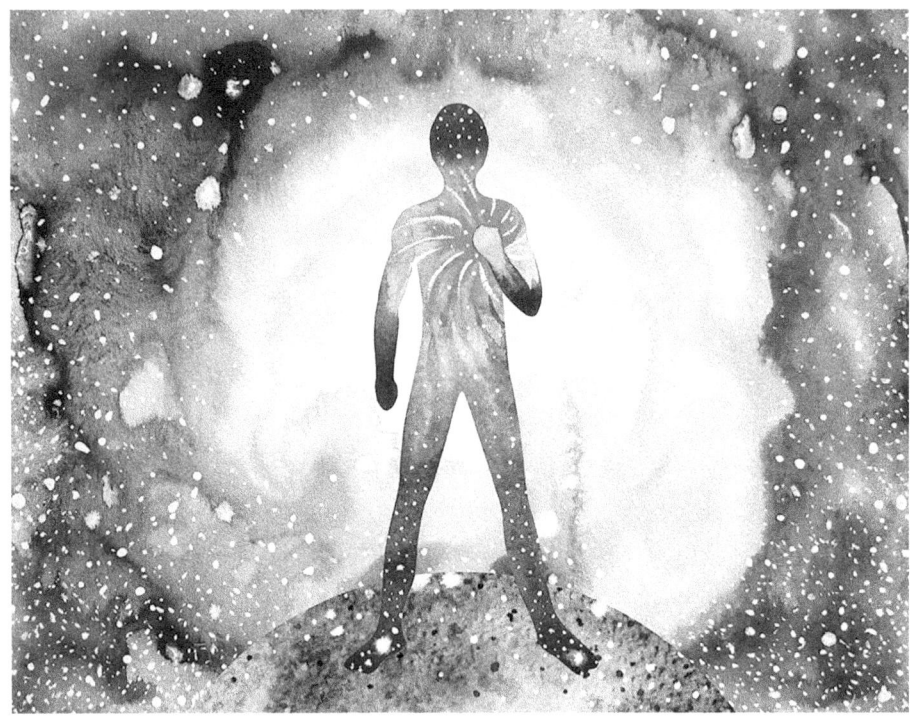

Power to the heart

What do we invest in and what do we empower?

Living from the heart is more than words, it requires commitment and fuel. It is something that can be cultivated and learned. It can help if we understand a little of the energetic heart's makeup and wisdom.

First off 'the heart knows' – start to acknowledge respect and value this wisdom a little more every day.

It is also the meeting place between heaven and earth so it is of itself balanced, it has no particular charge or volition to take sides. It is this absence of egoic charge that makes the heart so powerful.

Do not misunderstand, this is not nihilism, rather the very source of unconditional love.

1. **Prayer squats.** (a) Inhale – lift arms above head, palms together in prayer, legs slightly wider than hips, (b) exhale – squat down, keeping the torso vertical, then (c) smoothly bend forward from the waist bringing the hands to the floor. Then (d) inhale – straighten the legs keeping the hands on the ground. (e) exhale – return to the squatting position, hands on the ground, then smoothly (f) straighten up from the waist, arms raised, hands in prayer, then finally (g) inhale – straighten the knees and return to the original position. Keep repeating sequence, 3 min.

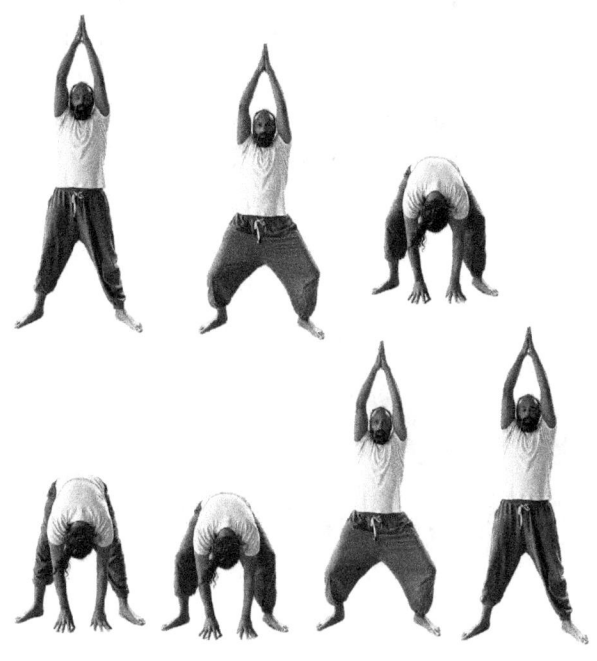

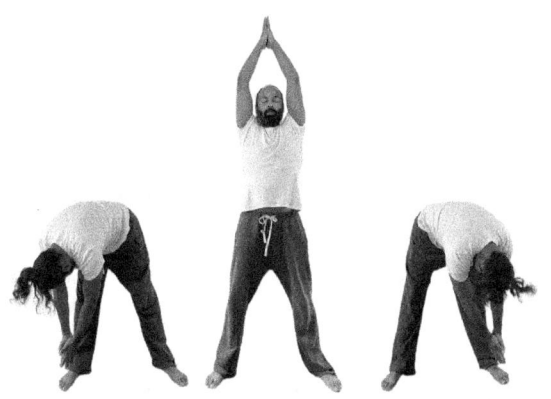

2. **Wide leg 'chop the wood'.** Inhale – stand with legs hip-width apart, arms straight and above the head, palms together. Exhale – bend from waist across left leg, keeping the torso and arms aligned in a 'chopping action'. Inhale back into the centre. Repeat across right leg, continue alternating between left and right legs. 3–5 min.

3. **Cat cow.** Come on to all fours, begin to flex the spine. Inhale as the spine arches downward and the head rises (cow). Exhale as the spine arches upward and the head releases down (cat). Move smoothly, gradually increasing the speed as the body opens. 2–3 min.

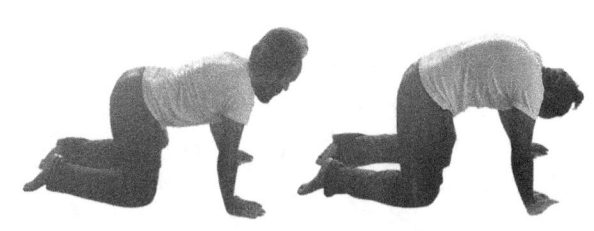

4. **Front platform 'knee ins'.** Come into a press-up position. Bring right knee towards left elbow and return. Bring right knee to the centre line of the chest and return. Bring right knee to right elbow and return. Repeat with left leg. Continue to alternate between right and left leg sequence. 2–3 min.

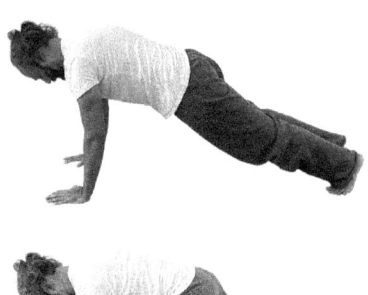

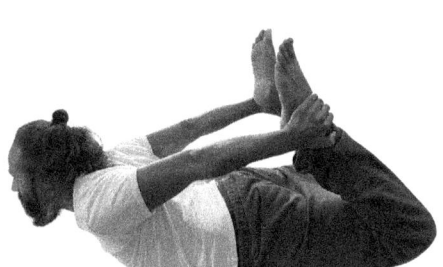

5. **Bow pose.** Lie on your front and grab hold of the ankles, lift the chest and aim to come up high while keeping the knees relatively narrow. Breath of fire, 1–3 min.

6. **Stretch pose.** Lie on the back, engage the core muscles of the stomach, bringing the lower back into the ground. Lift the legs up 15–30 cm, and the head up the same height and gaze at the toes, the arms come up the sides. Have a feel of lengthening (stretching) the body in this position, breath of fire. 2 min.

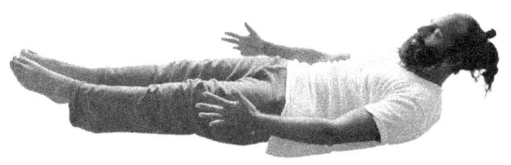

7. **Bear grip 5-5-5-5.** Sit in easy pose with bear grip, the right palm faces inwards about 15–20 cm away from the chest and clasps the fingers of the left hand, which faces away from the body. The elbows are out to the side. Face and shoulders relaxed, keep a gentle tension in the grip and keep the arms parallel to the ground.
Inhale for a count of 5 Hold breath for a count of 5 pull more strongly through the fingers.
Exhale for count of 5 reduce grip to normal levels.
Hold breath OUT for a count of 5 pull more strongly through fingers.

Repeat this sequence, 3–5 min.

8. **Spinal flex**. Sit cross-legged, hold on to the shins. Inhale as you move the spine forward, exhale as spine moves backwards. 1–3 min.

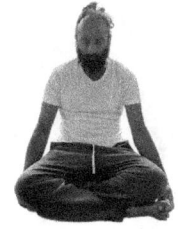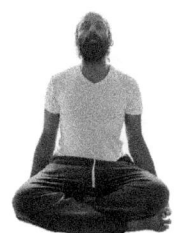

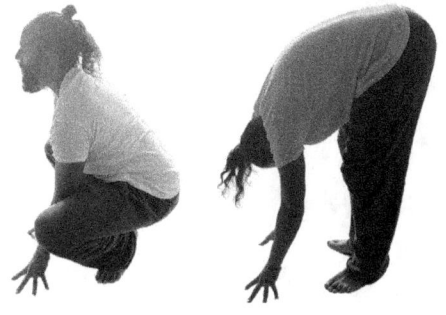

9. **Slow frogs**.
Come into a squatting position on the toes, heels together, hands together and fingertips on the ground. Inhale, slowly straighten the legs, allow torso neck and head to drop forward. Exhale slowly return to the original position. 1–2 min.

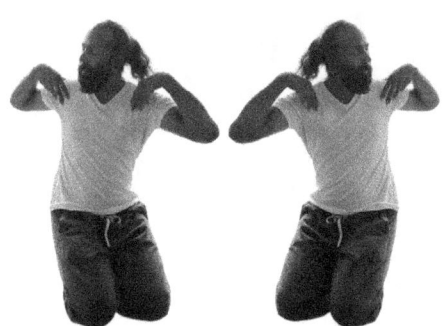

10. **On knees spinal twist**. Sit back on your heels in a kneeling position. Place hands on shoulders, inhale as you twist torso to left, exhale as you twist right. Move dynamically, 2–3 min.

11. **Pranayama sequence.** Inhale through left nostril, 2–3 min. Inhale through right nostril, 2–3 min.

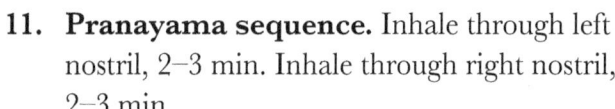

12. **Meditation** – Make a triangle shape with your index finger and thumbs, 5–8 cm in front of chest. Inhale long and deep, through an O-shaped mouth, visualising the prana of the breath entering through the triangle, directly into anahata chakra. Then chant the sound of the heart, 'Yam'(in long form Yaaaaaaaaammm), until you have no more breath. Repeat 3 min.

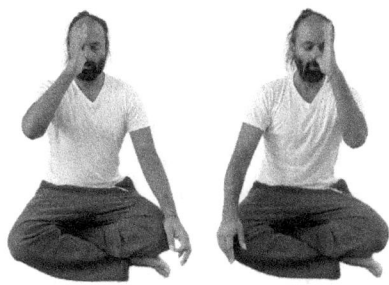

13. **Relax** –8–15 min

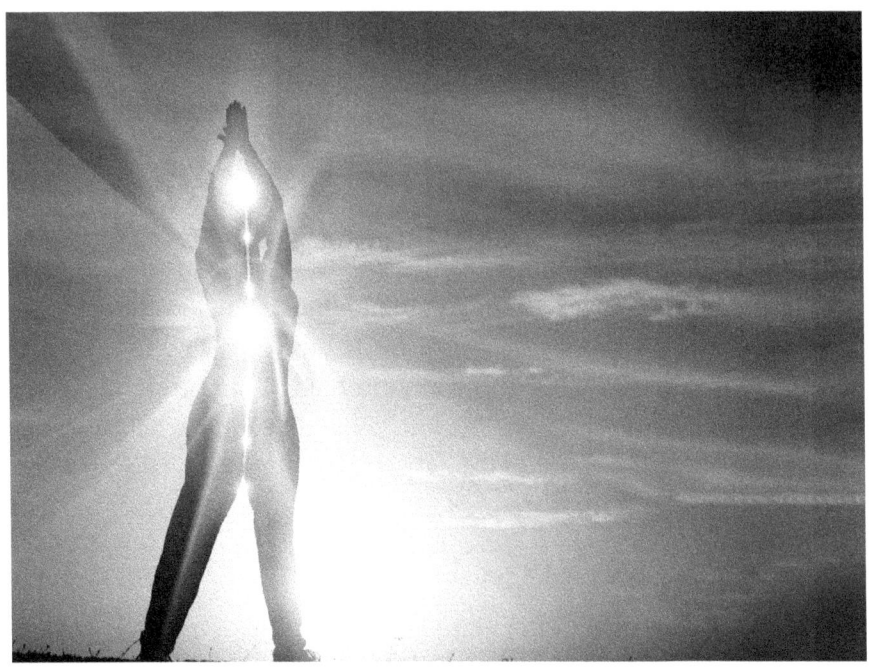

Standing steady in expansion – let it come to you

Steady sometimes gets a bad press; we tend to want shock and awe. Yet in our world I am afraid to say shock and awe often lack the substance to sustain, in time we learn to see the value of steady.

In fact when we look closely it gives all we want.

Steady in this context is the sun; it never fails. You can bet your house that that the sun shall rise the next day, and in the one-in-a-billion chance it does not you probably would have no need for a house anyway!

The sun illuminates and it gives constantly and steadily, yes clouds and wind may get in the way but the self-illuminated one is ever steady.

We just need to realise it and the clouds and winds of our life shall recede and we shall bask in the light of our illuminated self.

1. **On back quad stretch.** Lie on back legs out. Hug left knee into the chest and hold there with long deep breathing, right leg remains straight and relaxed on floor. Yield with each breath more deeply into the position. Switch sides after 1 min, then repeat.

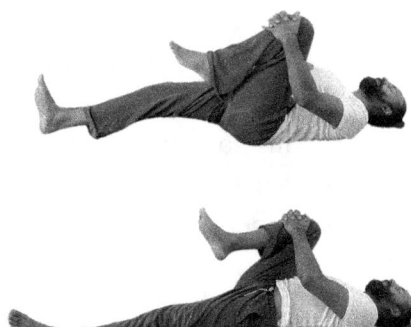

2. **On back knee rotations.** Hug both knees into the chest and rotate them in a circular direction massaging the lower back. 1 min one direction then change direction for a further minute.

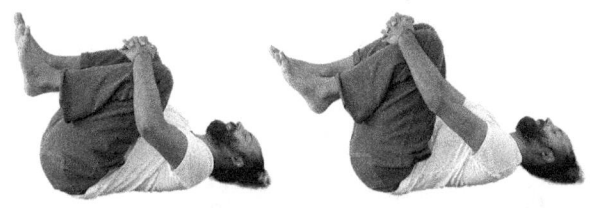

3. **Pelvic lifts – up and down.** Lie on back, knees up, soles of the feet on the ground, inhale and lift the pelvis off the ground, press strongly through legs and feet to lift pelvis. Exhale, lower back to the ground vertebrae by vertebrae. 1–3 min.

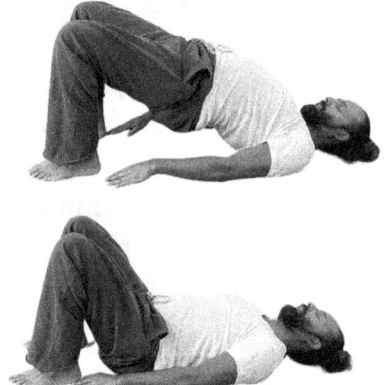

4. **Butterfly**. In a seated position hold the soles of the feet together, knees out to the side. Move the knees up and down in small movements like a 'butterfly'. Breathe long and deep. 1–3 min.

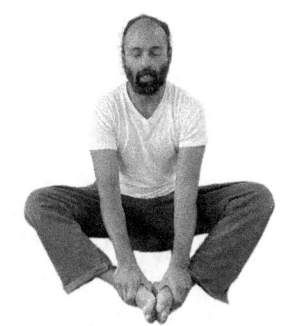

5. **Life nerve followed by hold with breath of fire.** Sit with the legs out straight, reach forward and grab the toes, in this position exhale and fold forward from the waist, inhale, return back up, move without forcing keeping the shoulders relaxed. Move quickly for 2–3 min.

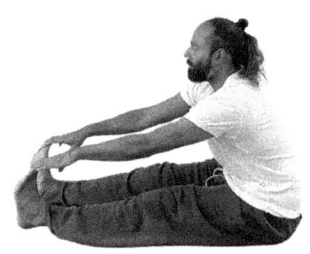

Inhale, hold the breath for 10 seconds. Then keep the extended position, this time without moving up and down, but keeping a strong lift out of the waist with the spine. Begin breath of fire. 1 min.

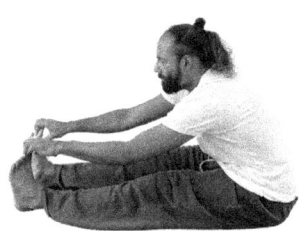

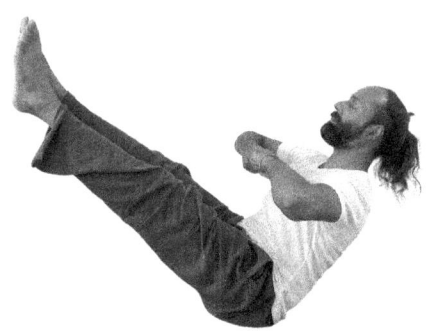

6. **Boat pose – with interlocked index fingers.** Sit with the legs straight and up at an angle of 60 degrees, the torso is at an equivalent angle. The index fingers are interlocked and pull against each other. Hold with breath of fire. 1–3 min.

7. **Archer pose lunges.** Stand and bring your right foot forward into a lunge bending at the knee, the left leg is straight with the foot extended out to the side at an angle of 45 degrees. The right arm is extended straight out parallel to the ground, the thumb of the right hand is extended with the fingers tucked into the top of the palm. The left hand is pulled into the left armpit, the image is of an archer aiming their bow.

Keeping this shape in mind, straighten and bend the right knee 1 min. Then for the final 2 minutes just hold the lunge position with long deep breathing. To finish, inhale and hold the breath for 10 seconds. Change sides and repeat the same process with the left foot forward.

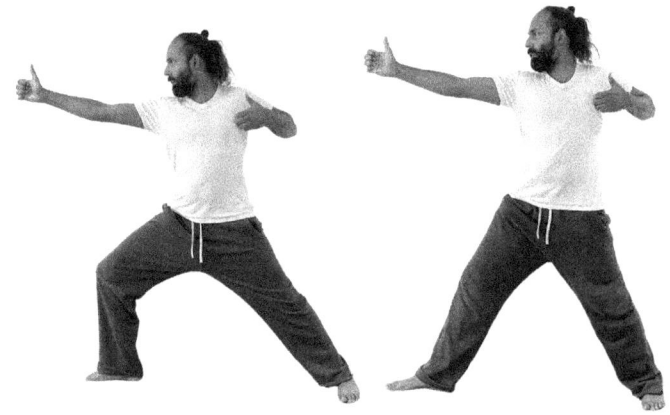

YOGA FOR FREEDOM

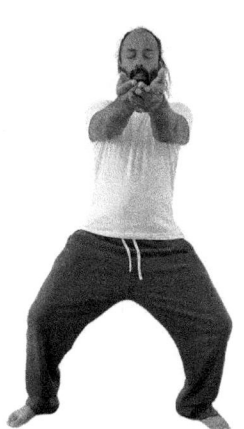

8. **Horse pose – catch the rain.** Stand with feet wider than the hips (the feet can angle a little outwards). Bend the knees and extend the arms straight, hands cupped. Breathe long and deep. 1.5–3 min.

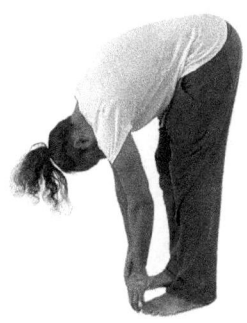

9. **Forward hang.** From a standing position feet hip-width apart (or closer if you prefer), fold from the waist keeping the legs as straight as possible for you. Hang here, release the head, neck and shoulders, breathe long and deep. 1.5–3 min.

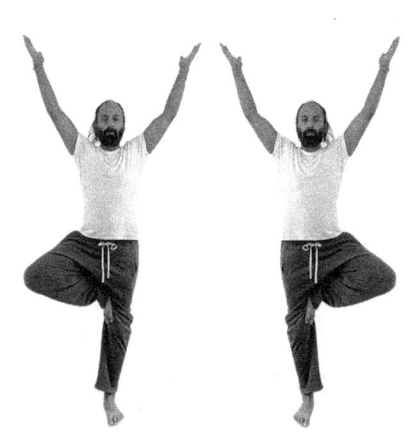

10. **Tree pose.** Stand straight, take a moment to ground yourself. Shift some of your weight on your right foot and then bring the sole of the left foot to rest against the inner right thigh. Bring the hands into prayer pose at the centre of the chest. To help keep balance focus on a point in the distance with relaxed eyes. Hold for 1 minute with long deep breathing, for last 30 seconds bring the arms up in a V shape with a slight opening of the chest. To finish, inhale and hold the breath for 5–10 seconds. Repeat the process for the opposite leg.

11. **Relax** – 10 min

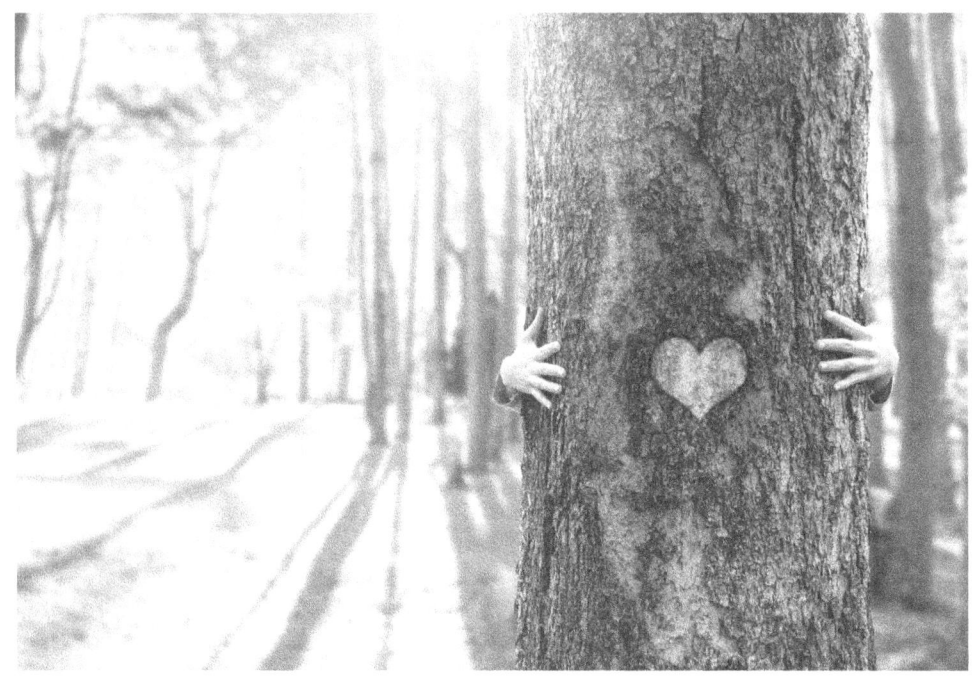

Embracing one's strength

Mind can slay you or make you.

When an army is scattered and spread thin it lacks cohesiveness and direction. It can be surrounded, or simply lack the power of a collective consciousness with the concept of self-direction.

The subconscious mind has the habit of taking us on a journey of projections or misunderstandings – defining our self in relation to others or our culture. Like a disjointed army, we become scattered fighting on multiple fronts against a fictional enemy.

Embracing one's strength is like ordering an army to stop fighting a false enemy, relinquish their weapons and come home.

As our 'intention energy' returns to us; by simply disengaging our mind, we accomplish something quite spectacular. We ignite our inner power and strength. We realise the illusion and we become a unified force – illuminated and at peace with ourselves there is no need for war.

1. **Hug the body throw the water.** In a seated position, arms relaxed, inhale, bring the elbows back past the ribs; exhale, hug the torso. Inhale, arms back, elbows past the ribs. Inhale, throw the forearm and hands back, passed the shoulders. Inhale, elbows back; exhale, hug the torso (changing the cross of the arms). Keep going like this 2–3 min.

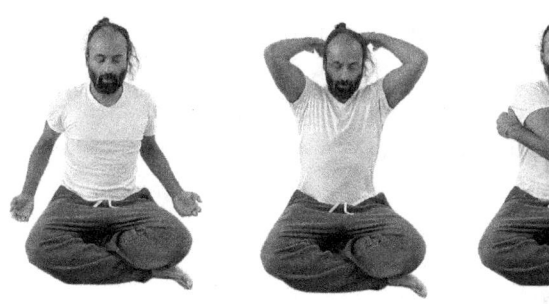

2. **Arms out finger pulses.** Remain seated arms straight out to the side, fingers outstretched, bring the fingers into the top part of the palm and release them back out quickly. Time the movement with breath of fire. 3–5 min.

3. **On knees spinal flex.** Sit in a kneeling position. Hands on thighs, inhale flex spine forward, exhale flex backwards. Eyes closed focussed on brow. 2–3 min.

4. **Warrior dog.** Come into a downward dog, keeping the downward dog shape, lower yourself down by bending your arms (like a press-up), then begin to transition into upward-facing dog by moving into a plank-like position and then straightening the arms and opening the chest into cobra. 1–3 min.

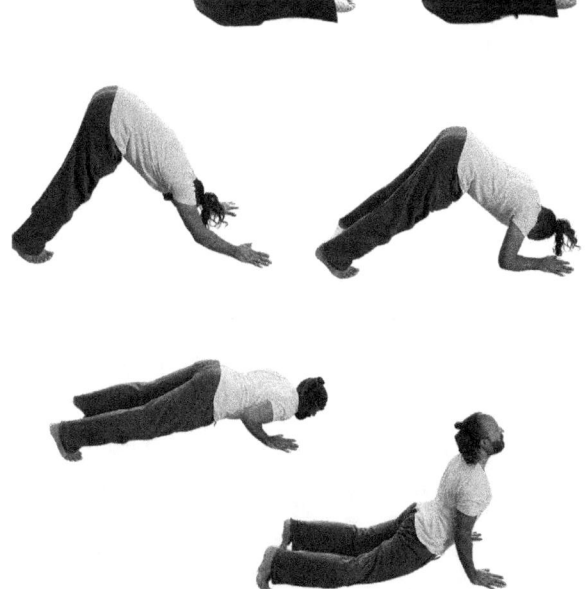

5. **Bow pose 5-5-5.** Lie on your front and grab hold of the ankles, lift the chest and aim to rise up across the inhale for a count of 5. Hold the breath and the bow position for a count of 5. Exhale down across a count of 5. Repeat this sequence 2–3 min.

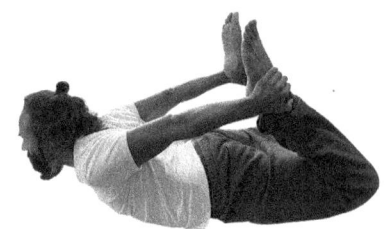

6. **Front platform on forearms – interlaced fingers.** Come on to the forearms, interlacing the fingers, legs out straight behind you resting on the toes. Hold this position with breath of fire, 1–2 min.

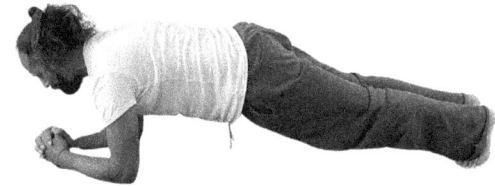

7. **Rocking bow.** Lie on your front and grab hold of the ankles, lift the chest and hold the position with long deep breathing, allowing the body to come into a natural rocking motion.

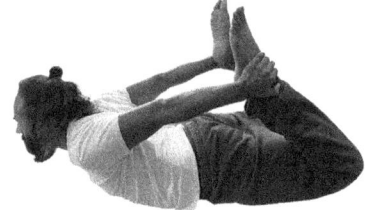

8. **Lie on back arms and legs up 90 degrees.** Lie on back, raise up arms, shoulder-width apart, fingers to ceiling, palms facing. Legs raised 90 degrees. Breathe 2–3 min.

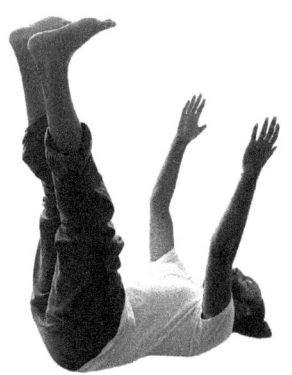

9. **Frogs.** Come into a squatting position on the toes, heels together, hands together and fingertips on the ground. Inhale, straighten the legs, allow torso neck and head to drop forward. Exhale, return to the original position. 1–2 min.

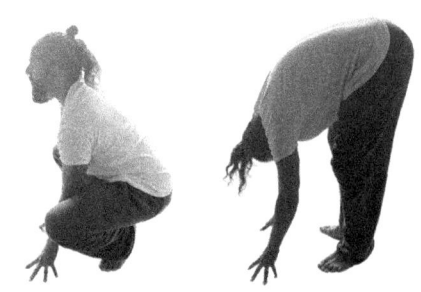

10. **Swirl the torso.** Come standing on the knees, arms up, start to rotate the upper shoulders and arms in a devotional manner changing the direction occasionally. Continue 1–3 min.

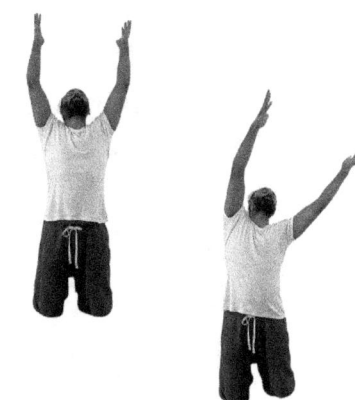

11. **Tree pose.** Come standing, find a point in the distance to focus on for balance, bring the right foot into the inner left thigh. Hands at centre of chest in prayer pose, and when balance is stable, open the arms up and out like the canopy of a tree. Hold this position for a count of 10 long deep breaths. Then change sides and repeat.

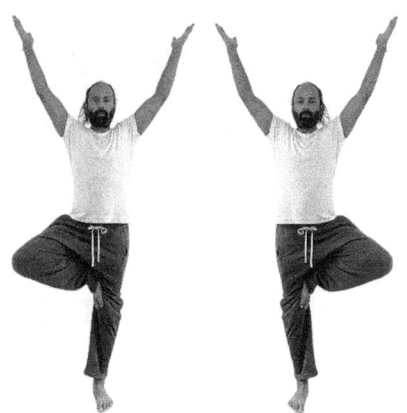

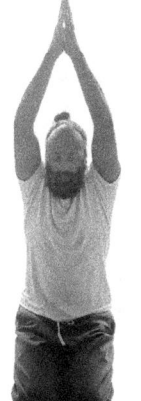

12. **On knees arms extended chant 'Hari Nam'*.** Sitting back on heels, arms extended above, head straight, palms together in a prayer pose, start to chant the mantra, '**Hari, Hari, Hari, Hari, Hari, Hari, Hari, Naam**'. Drawing in on the navel on Hari.

<u>Hari</u> – Divinity uttered to take away negativity – one Hari for each of the 7 chakras.

<u>Naam</u> – A dedication in reverence – presented into the aura.

Bring the light – preparing the body for soul action

Light can express itself as a wave and a particle, that's how cool it is. For the second phenomenon to arise it requires awareness. Some observer or witness to create the potential for the co-creation of some reality?

Light one could say is the fuel for our creation but it needs an architect. The more conscious the architect, the more profound and powerful the light display. The energy of light is at the source of our being. It is in our cells, if we are able to harness it we become like generators. The vibration somehow emitting a frequency that can be sensed by others.

If we understand that light is that which is the true fuel for our actions and that the quality of its vibration matters then we can become increasingly aware of its qualities and nuances. One of its most beautiful offerings is joy. So come bring the light, bring the joy and 'boss it'.

1. **Shiva run.** Run on the spot, arms up, palms face forward held at right angles. Run and keep the knees up. Run with joy and vigour, knees up. 3–11 min.

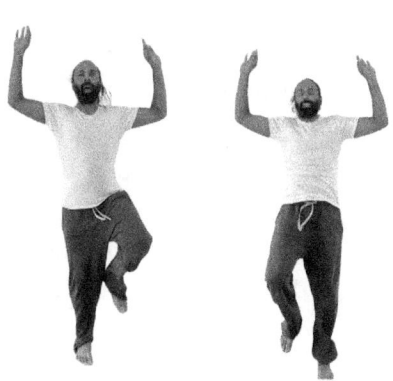

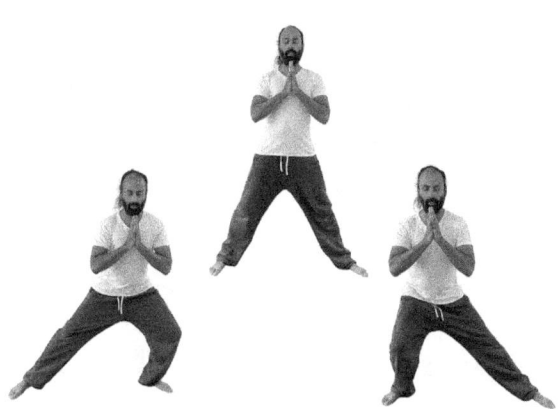

2. **Dancing Goddess side to side.** Come into goddess pose, legs wider than hips, hands in prayer at the centre of the chest. Inhale, straddle to the left. Exhale back to the middle, inhale, straddle to the right. Keep moving smoothly & rhythmically between left and right positions. Open to the goddess energy. 2–3 min.

3. **Standing wide leg life nerve.** Keeping the legs wide and straight, bring the arms up above the head straight, palms facing the ceiling. Inhale. Exhale, fold from the waist, bring the hands towards the floor. 1–3 min.

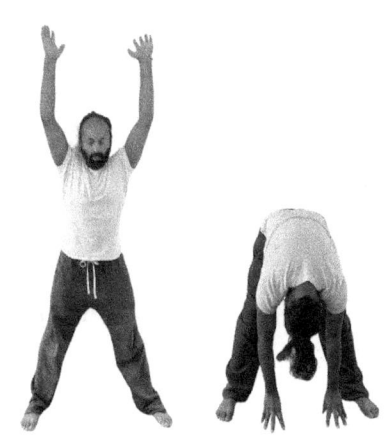

4. **On knees torso twist.** Come on to the knees. Sit tall, hands interlaced behind your back, arms straight. Begin to twist the torso left and right. Inhale left, exhale right. 1–3 min.

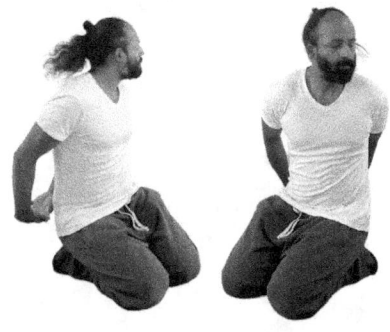

5. **8-stroke eagle wings**. On knees, with the arms straight and fingertips just touching the ground either side of the hips. Inhale in 8 strokes through the nose while smoothly moving the arms up keeping them straight, at the end of the eighth stroke the backs of the hands touch. Then smoothly bring the arms down as you complete eight strokes out. At the end of the eighth stroke out, your hands are back in the original position. Fingers touching the ground. 2–5 min.

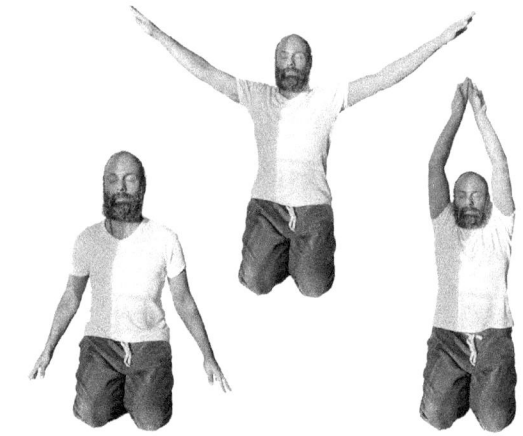

6. **Swirl the torso.** Stand on knees, raise arms overhead, begin to rotate arms and upper torso in circles with devotion. 2–4 min.

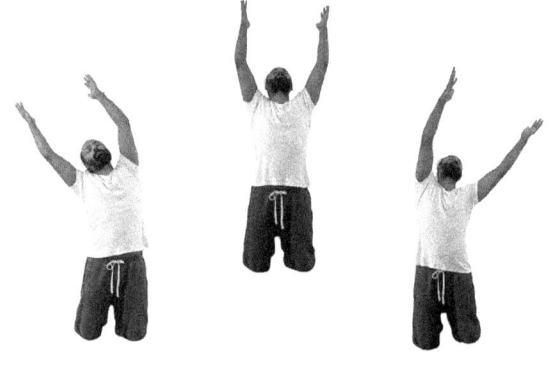

7. **Gurpranam.** Bring the forehead to the ground and sit back on the heels. Reach out along the ground with the arms bringing the palms together into prayer pose. Rest here with long deep breathing. 2–3 min.

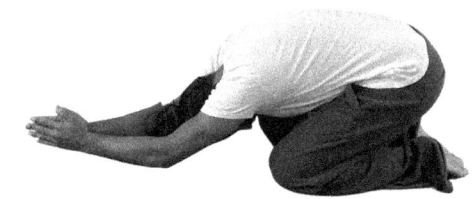

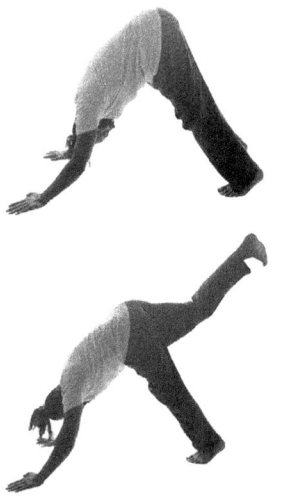

8. **Downward dog leg march.** On all fours, knees beneath hips, hands beneath shoulders, lift the buttocks off the ground coming on to the toes. Straighten the legs creating a triangular shape with the body. Rest in this position for 30 sec – 1 min. Then in this position begin to march the legs up and down keeping them straight, inhale as the right leg comes up, exhale as it goes down. Inhale as the left leg rises, exhale as it goes down. 1.5–3 min.

9. **Chant 'Shakyamuni mantra'** – **Om Muni Muni Maha Muniye Shakyamuni Soha.* 5–11 min.

10. **Shavasana** – 5–11 min

> Shakyamuni mantra is said to reference the ancestral tribe of the Buddha. The words revere the great sage from this tribe (the Buddha) who shared the wisdom of enlightenment. For me chanting this mantra is powerfully devotional and relatable. He was a human being who became enlightened and then shared their light. May the chain continue.

🎧 Music suggestion: Shakyamuni mantra by Manish Vyas

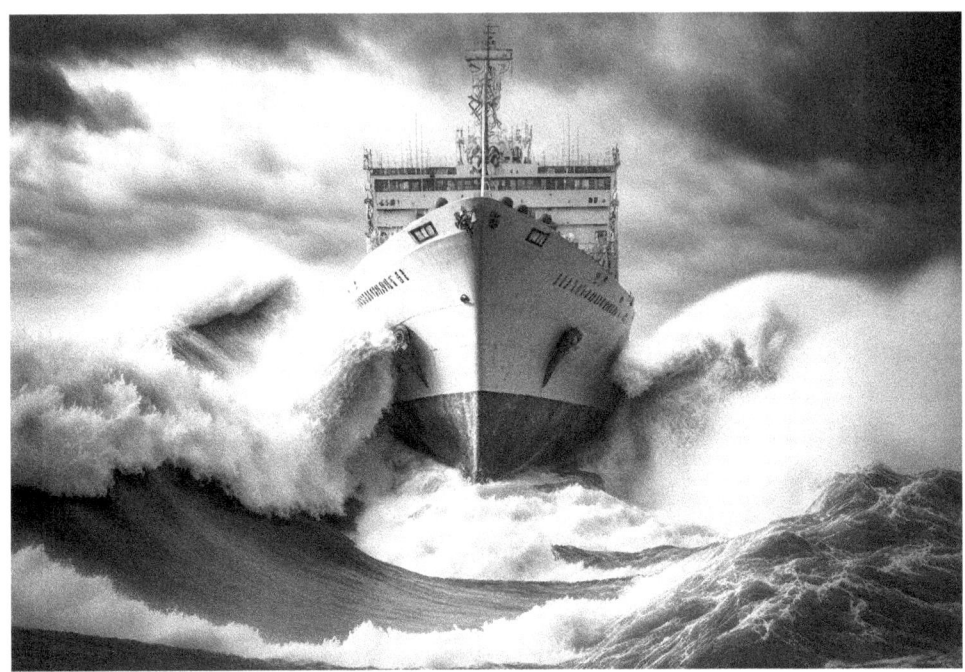

Steady the ship

When the metaphorical ship starts to shake or rock. We have a choice, we either embrace calamity or equanimity.

Calamity amplifies, doubling up on wavelengths of fear and worry.

Equanimity reaches into our reserves, draws upon our grit and fires up our wise focus. It counteracts the movements of polarity through anchoring in singularity.

It also asks us to widen our perception and see holistically what is playing out as unstable waters.

Taking a too-narrow view can lead us to see the problem two-dimensionally.

If, however, we can bring in more space, the turbulence almost always lessens, it's as if we immediately reduce the anxiety and the constriction that often brings.

1. **Standing squats.** Standing feet hip-width apart (or a little wider). Fingers interlaced and placed behind head. Exhale, squat down; inhale, rise back up to the original position. 1–2 min.

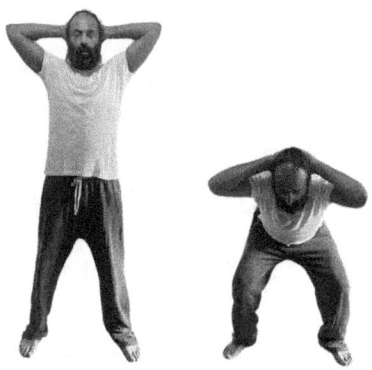

2. **Windmills**. Stand with legs wide, arms out to the side, reach through fingers, anchor through the legs. Spine lifted, inhale. Exhale, right hand moves towards left foot. Inhale, return back to the original position. Exhale, left hand moves to right foot. Keep moving, smoothly with awareness and full of breathing. 2–3 min.

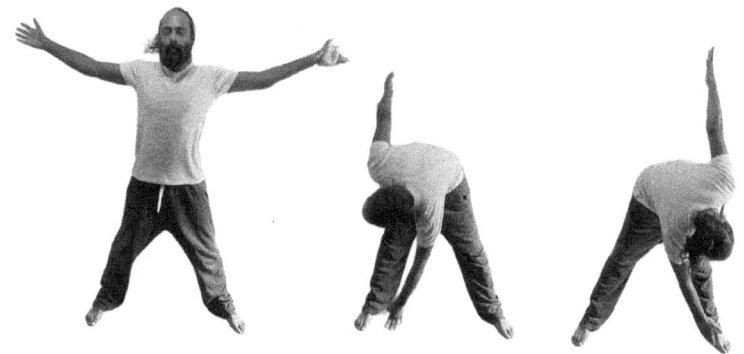

3. **Standing torso twists/arm flails.** Standing straight, feet hip-width apart. Keep arms very relaxed, turn torso left and right, allowing the arms to start to move around the body in a relaxed manner. 1–2 min.

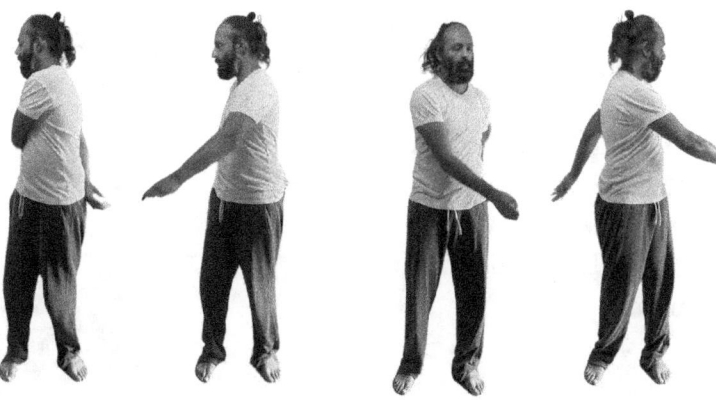

4. **Standing side stretch**. Stand with feet hip-width apart. Inhale, reach the right arm up and arch across above the head while grounding strongly through the right leg. Exhale as you come back through the middle smoothly moving to the opposite side (left arm arcs up to the right while anchoring the left leg). Keep moving smoothly in this manner. 2–3 min.

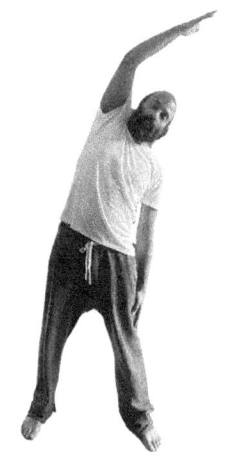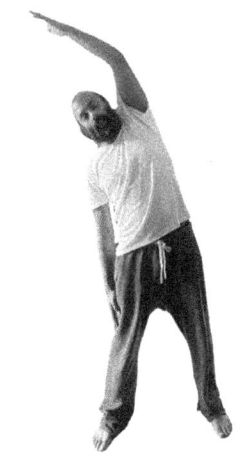

5. **Life nerve**. Sit with the legs out straight, reach forward and grab the toes, in this position exhale and fold forward from the waist, inhale, return back up, move without forcing, keeping the shoulders relaxed. Move quickly 2–3 min.

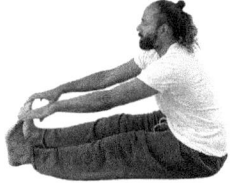

6. **Pranayama sequence**

Seated in easy pose.
- Block right nostril with right thumb. Inhale and exhale through left nostril. Repeat 1–3 min.
- Block left nostril with left thumb. Inhale and exhale through right nostril. Repeat 1–3 min.
- Block right nostril with right thumb, inhale through left nostril. Release the right nostril, block the left nostril with little finger of right hand, exhale through right nostril. Repeat this breathing pattern. 1–3 min.
- Block left nostril with left thumb, inhale through right nostril. Release the left nostril, block the right nostril with little finger of left hand, exhale through left nostril. Repeat this breathing pattern. 1–3 min.

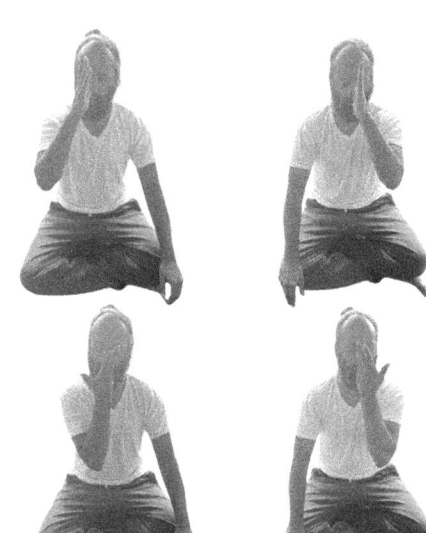

7. **X shape on ground.** Lie on the back, form an X shape with your body. Begin breath of fire in this position. 1–3 min.

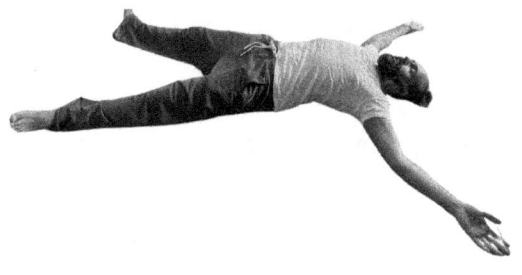

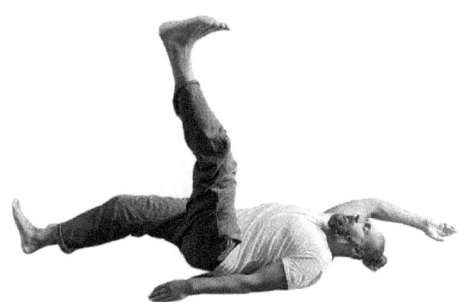

8. **March on back**. Lie on back, inhale, left leg rises up, at the same time bring up right arm. Exhale, return left leg and right arm back to the ground. Inhale, lift right leg and left arm. Keep moving like this. 2–3 min.

9. **Double leg lifts.** Remain on back, inhale, lift both legs up to 90 degrees. Exhale, return the legs back to the ground.

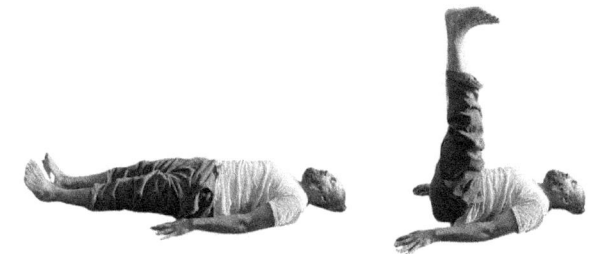

10. **Half wheel.** Lie on back, knees up, soles of feet on ground. Press through the feet to lift the pelvis off the ground. Hold elevated position and begin breath of fire. 2–3 min.

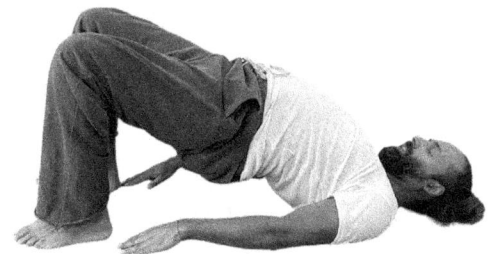

11. **Bounce, move, dance on back**. Lie on the back and start to move randomly, fluidly, intuitively, dynamically, hips, shoulders, feet head, etc. Just move and release. Continue 1–2 min.

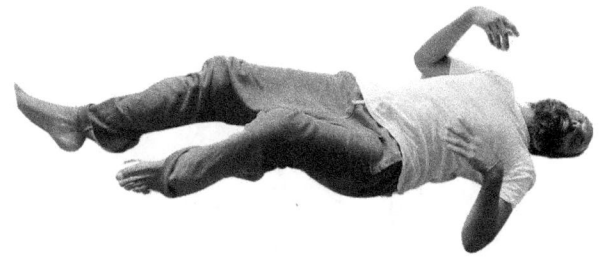

12. Chant **Maha Mrityunjaya mantra, 108 recitation or 5–30 mins.**

> **Maha Mrityunjaya mantra** is said to have a range of applications. But in my experience is especially powerful when something challenging lands in your life – it may be a nice one to use. Often chanted 108 times.
>
> Om Tryambhakam Yajamahe
> Sugandhim Pushtivardhanam
> Urvarukamiva Bandhanan
> Mrityor Mukshiya Maamritat

🎧 Music suggestion: Maha Mrityunjaya by Ketan Patwardhan

13. **Shavasana** 5–11 min.

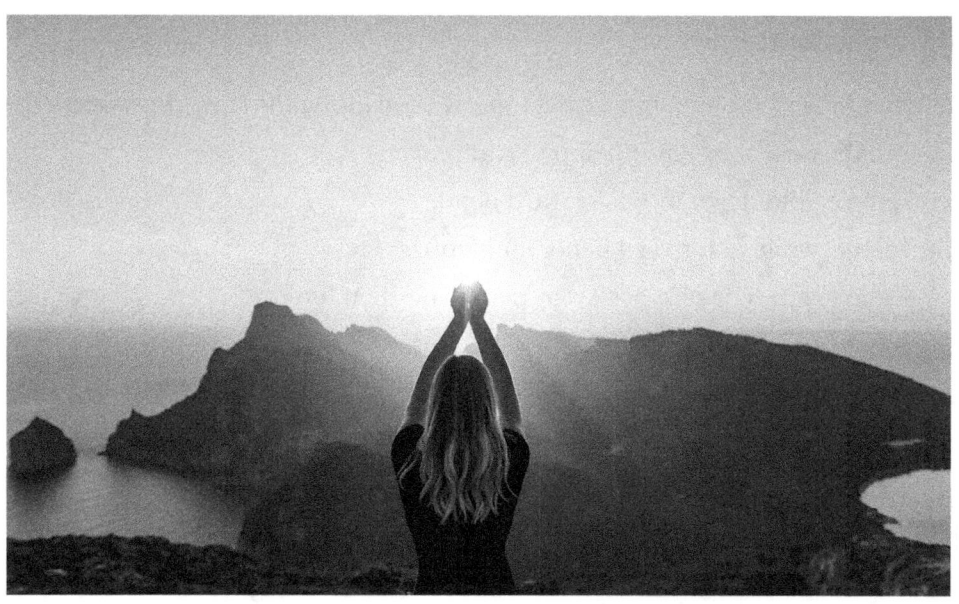

Passion for Divine

How we decide to use our life force is a question of prime importance, at a time where our attention and intention can be exponentially scattered.

The dispersion of our vitality and concentrated mind can seriously deplete our effectiveness, impact and happiness. All are interconnected and feed into our primary drive to live in alignment with a sense of purposefulness.

We must counteract the tendency to disperse, that is, to have our focus pulled in a million directions so we end up achieving nothing of substance, we end up following the curated agendas of culture and become open to our sense of self being hijacked.

One of the most simple and powerful remedies to counteract the pull into duality is to invest in unity.

It is effective as you don't have to hunt down all your missing parts, you simply return to that which was always there?!

1. **3-5 sun salutations**

    a. Standing in mountain pose, feet together, arms by the side, chest open.
    b. Inhale, raise the arms up above into prayer.
    c. Exhale, fold down into a forward bend.
    d. Inhale, while in forward bend, look up.
    e. Exhale, jump or step back into plank and then lower down to the ground.
    f. Inhale, upward-facing dog.
    g. Exhale, downward-facing dog, 5 breaths.
    h. Inhale, jump or step forward into a forward bend and look up.
    i. Exhale, drop the head down into the forward bend.
    j. Inhale, rise into standing bring arms up above head, hands touch in prayer.
    k. Exhale, arms come down to sides, stand in mountain pose.

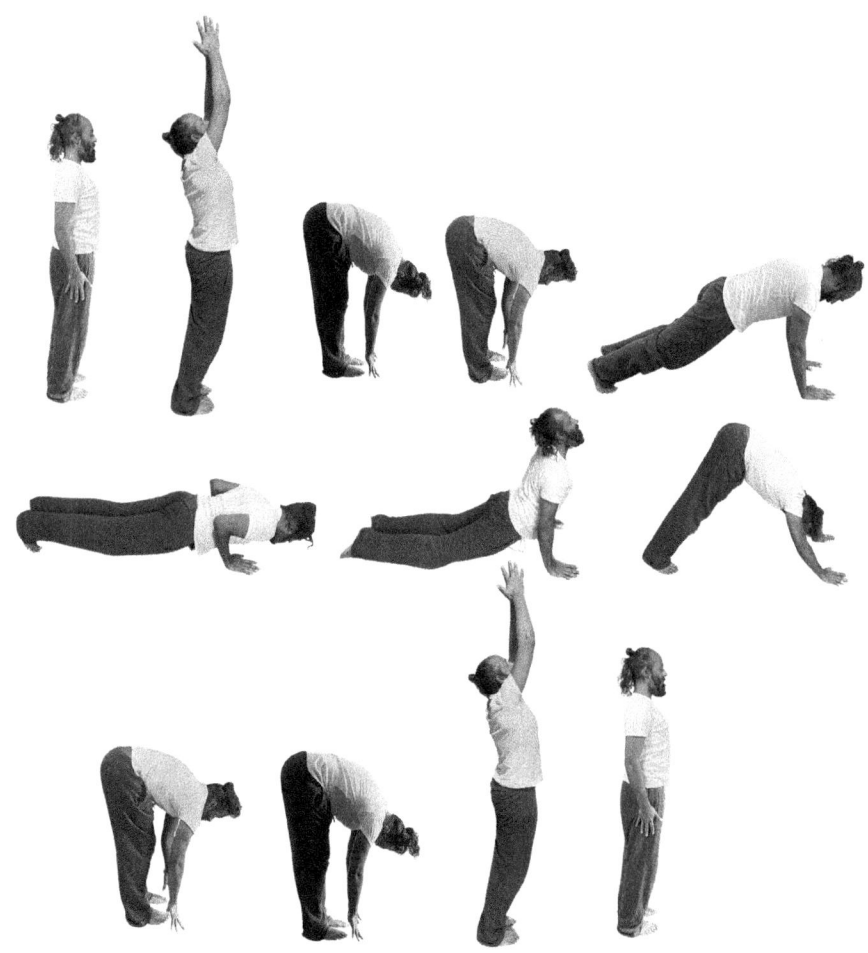

2. **Slow miracle bends.** Feet hip-width apart, arms up, palms face the ceiling, a sense of an open chest. Exhale and move the hands to the ground, keeping the arms extended. Inhale, return to the original position. Move with awareness. The movement is not overly quick. Continue 2–3 min.

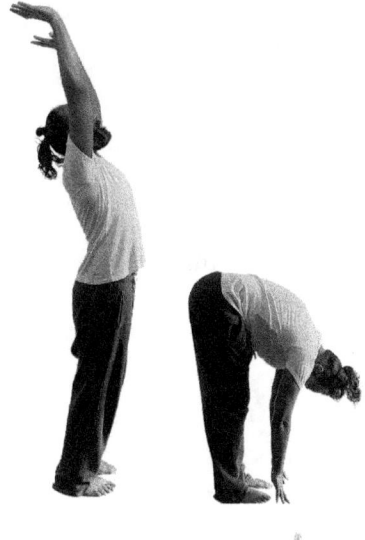

3. **Potency hold knees 1–2 min, followed by arms up hands in prayer.** Heels together, bend the knees slightly. Press the muscles either side of the knees with the thumb and the fingers. Relax and hold this position, but keep a sense of elevation and lift out of the base of the spine. Eyes closed or slightly open keeping focus on a point in the distance. 1–2 min.

Keeping the same body position just change the arms, bring them up and extend them above the head, palms together, arms long and aligned to the angle of torso. 1–2 min.

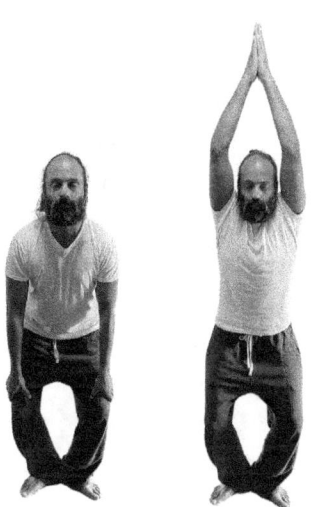

4. **Frogs**. Come into a squatting position on the toes, heels together, hands together and fingertips on the ground. Inhale, straighten the legs allow torso neck and head to drop forward. Exhale, return to the original position. 1–2 min.

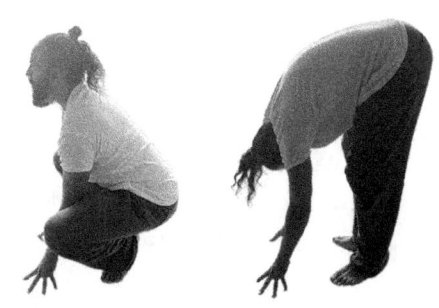

5. **Maha mudra.** Sit with your left heel in the perineum and right leg extended straight out. Reach forward, press the fleshy part of the big toe (if you can reach). Inhale, then exhale all the breath out. Apply all the bandhas and keep the breath held out for approximately 8 seconds. Continue 1–4 min. Then change sides and repeat the process for a further 1–4 min.

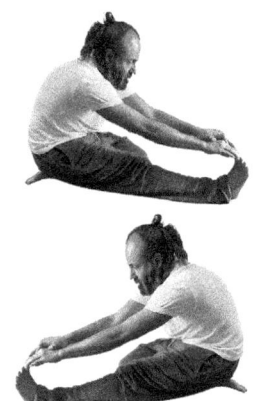

6. **Gurpranam to flower – *Music Sri Ram**. Sit back on heels, reach along the ground palms together. Play some devotional music, moving smoothly and devotionally come to a kneeling position, hands in prayer at the chest before smoothly coming up off the knees and extend up the arms before finally opening the arms wide at the end of the cycle, like a flower opening. Then reverse the movement, closing the flower down, returning to kneeling and finally back to gurpranam. Continue to repeat this movement in rhythm to the devotion mantra. Allow yourself to drop deep into the movement. 3–11 min.

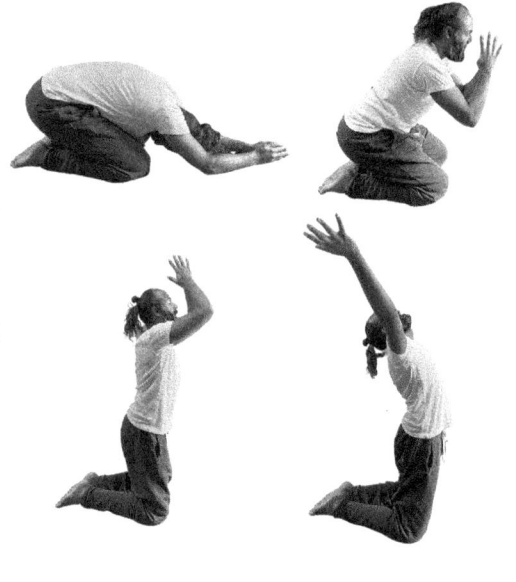

7. **Crossed arm leg lifts.** Lie on the back, cross arms at the chest. Rest here for 1 min, then inhale, lift the left leg up to 90 degrees, exhale, return the leg down. Inhale, lift the right leg up to 90 degrees, exhale down. Keep moving dynamically in this manner. 2–3 min. To finish, inhale, hold the breath, extend both legs straight at an angle of 60-degree hold for 10 seconds, before exhaling. Repeat this end sequence twice more.

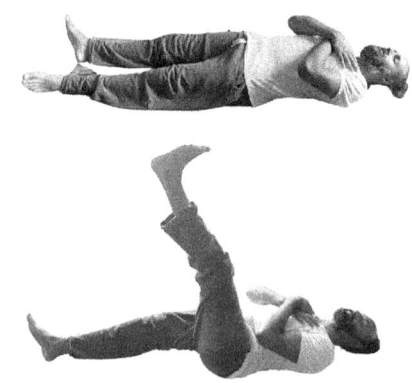

8. **On back cover ears move like a fish in the ocean.** Lie on back, legs straight and together, cover ears, elbows point to the ceiling. Move the hips side to side while keeping the remainder of body relaxed. Continue to move, go deep like into a trance. 2–3 min.

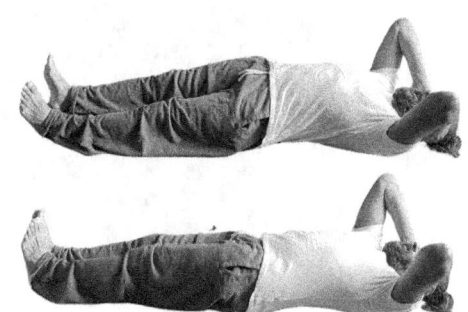

9. **Relax** 1 min.

10. **Fish pose.** Lie on the back, arms reach under the body, hands beneath buttocks / upper thighs. Raise up on the forearms (arms bearing all the weight), allow the chest to open and release the head back to the floor. Ensuring the arms are strong and stable – breathe long and deep. 30–60 seconds.

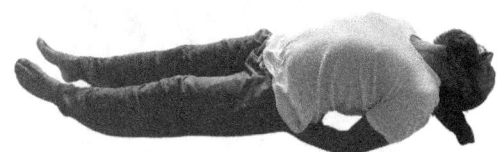

11. **Chant – *'Om Namah Shivaya'** 5–31 min

12. **Savasana** – 11 min

🎧 Music suggestion: Sri Ram and Om Nama Shivaya by Shantala

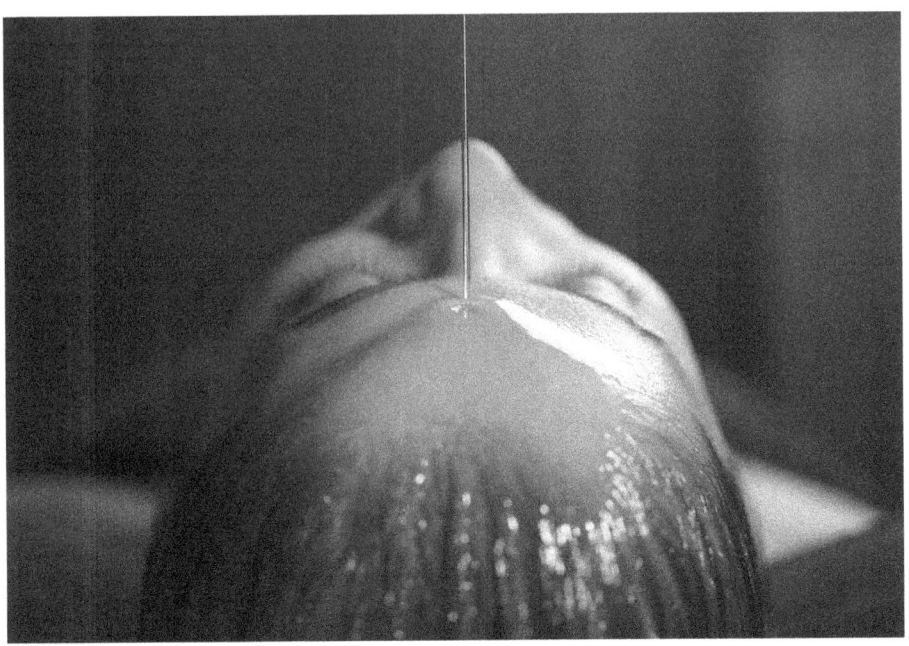

Clean out!

Claim your space in life.

We are holistic beings, finely balanced and we need to open to the flow of continual renewal to feel aligned and purposeful. However, we can overlook the need to clean out the old. It's like painting without first preparing the surface. At first nothing is seen but soon the karmic effect of the poor groundwork makes it to the surface.

When we don't clean out, we feel its effects literally under the skin (that dodgy paint job again), and if we don't deal with it like a clogged drain it backs up, until you are forced to. By that time, the fallout can be troublesome indeed, affecting our relationships, health and more.

So when you feel the first remnants of that build-up clogging up the space of your life, it's time to claim it back, by cleaning out the old. The body, emotions and energy system are deeply intertwined; yoga can access the energy streams that are blocked, cleaning, clearing and alleviating.

All supported by a powerful intention to clear.

1. **Punching.** Seated in easy pose, start to punch with relaxed fists. Allowing the torso to naturally twist left right as you punch with power, relaxation and rhythm. Inhale left, exhale right. 2–3 min.

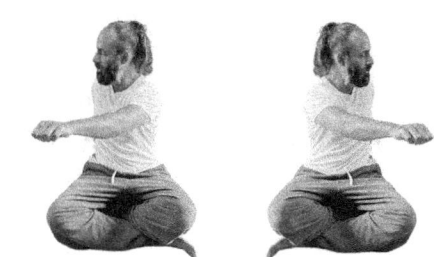

2. **Butt kicking.** Lie on back, begin to kick the buttocks with your heels (or get them as close as), exhaling as heel strike buttocks, move quickly. 2–3 min.

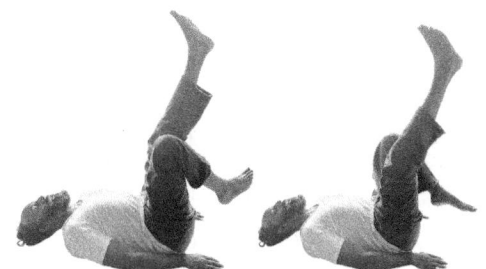

3. **Piston kicking.** Lie on back; engage core abdominal muscles, piston kick the legs by drawing one knee in towards the chest as the opposite leg extends straight around 30 cm above the ground. Breathe powerfully in rhythm to the motion. Move quickly so that the breath becomes almost like a breath of fire. 2–3 min.

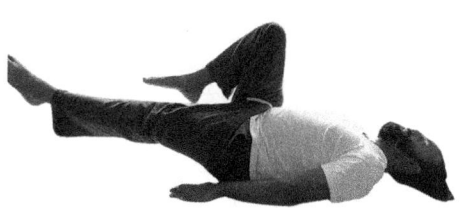

4. **Half wheel.** Lie on back, knees up, soles of feet on ground. Press through the feet to lift the pelvis off the ground. Hold elevated position and begin breath of fire. 2–3 min.

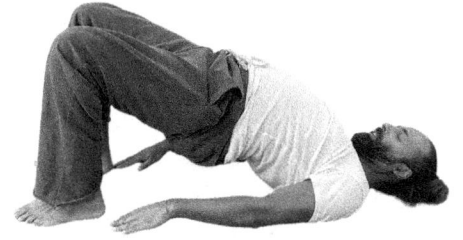

5. **Kick into forward bend.** Hug knees into chest, then exhale, dynamically kick legs out along the ground, at the same time the torso rises up into a forward bend, hands to toes. Inhale and return to the original position. Keep moving like this. 2–3 min.

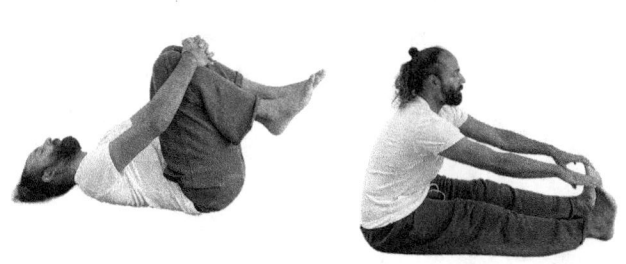

6. **On knees eagle wings O breath.** Sit on heels, arms out to the side, raise them up like eagles' wings with power and grace, powerful O-breath with mouth in rhythm to the movement. 2–5 min.

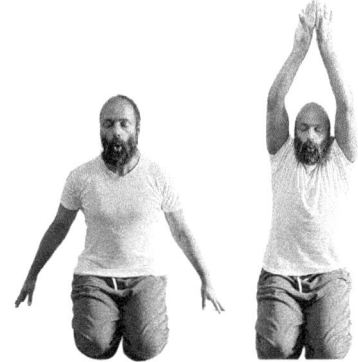

7. **Bow pose.** Lie on your front and grab hold of the ankles, lift the chest and breathe long and deep, allow a natural rocking motion to happen in rhythm to the breath. 1–3 min.

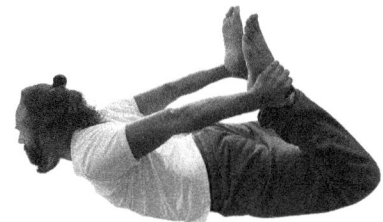

8. **Cobra – lion breath**. Lie on front, hands either side of shoulders, inhale. Push up into a Cobra. Inhale & Exhale through the mouth over an extended tongue (lion breath). 2–3 min.

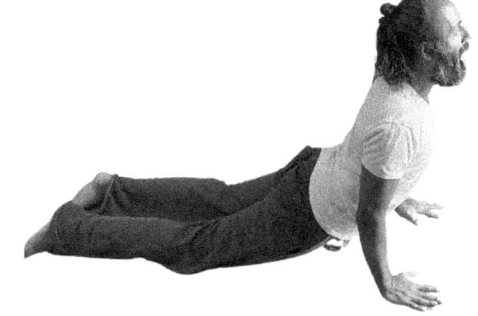

9. **Frogs 1–2 min**. Come into a squatting position on the toes, heels together, hands together and fingertips on the ground. Inhale, straighten the legs, allow torso neck and head to drop forward. Exhale, return to the original position. 1–2 min.

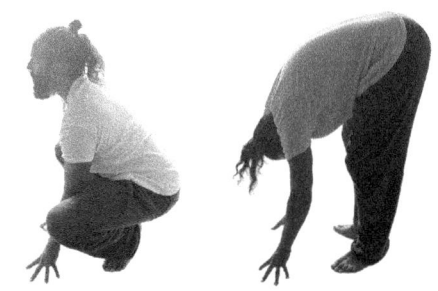

10. **Shavasana** 5–11 min

11. Chant '**Om Benza Satto Hung**' 5–31 min.

12. **Om Benza Satto Hung** – Highly vibrational mantra that works from the inside out at a cellular level.

🎧   Music suggestion: **Om Benza Satto Hung by Deval Premal and the Gyuto Monks of Tibet**

CONCLUSION

Practicing kriyā takes us on a journey of personal discovery.

We can respect, appreciate and even love kriyās for their effectiveness in elevating our frequency and for opening vistas of higher perception and healing.

Yet in that journey let us not forget the destination.

Leela presents so many expressions while our final destination remains the same, to come home to ourselves.

In our world of so much opportunity we may lose ourselves in the delight and travails of our journey. In the heights of peak experience and in the valleys of despair, remember that the true absolute reality never left you.

If you need a barometer for your practice let it be for peace in your life.

Leela will draw you into polarities that can be so subtle; true peace has no polarity and when you land there anything is possible.

ABOUT THE AUTHOR

Sivaroshan is of Sri Lankan Tamil descent. His grandparents immigrated from Sri Lanka to Malaysia and his parents from Malaysia to England. Born in the UK, he spent his formative years in North London and Essex.

Following higher education and travels, Sivaroshan pursued a career in the corporate sector. This dovetailed with an ever-deepening spiritual inquiry. His path led him to a vast array of spiritual explorations in the fields of meditation, energy healing and yoga.

You can find out more about Sivaroshan and his work at sivaroshan.co.uk.

www.ingramcontent.com/pod-product-compliance
Lightning Source LLC
LaVergne TN
LVHW081355060426
835510LV00013B/1827